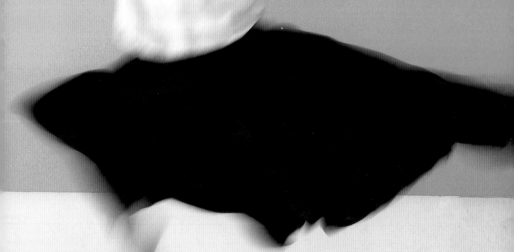

PERSONAL TRAINER
YOGA FOR KIDS

THIS IS A CARLTON BOOK

Text copyright © 2003 Liz Lark
Design and special photography copyright © 2003
Carlton Books Limited

This paperback edition published in 2010
by Carlton Books Limited
20 Mortimer Street
London W1T 3JW

10 9 8 7 6 5 4 3 2 1

ISBN 978 1 84732 668 3

Printed and bound in China

In the interest of good health, it is always important to consult your
doctor before commencing any exercise programme, especially if
you have a medical condition or are pregnant. All guidelines and
warnings should be read carefully.

The author and publisher have made every effort to ensure that
all information is correct and up to date at the time of publication.
Neither the author nor the publisher can accept responsibility for,
or shall be liable for, any accident, injury, loss or damage (including
any consequential loss) that results from using the ideas, information,
procedures or advice offered in this book.

Editorial Manager: Judith More

Art Director: Penny Stock

Senior Art Editor: Barbara Zuñiga

Executive Editor: Zia Mattocks

Design: DW Design

Editor: Lisa Dyer

Special photography: Clare Park

Stylist: Clare Park

Production: Janette Burgin

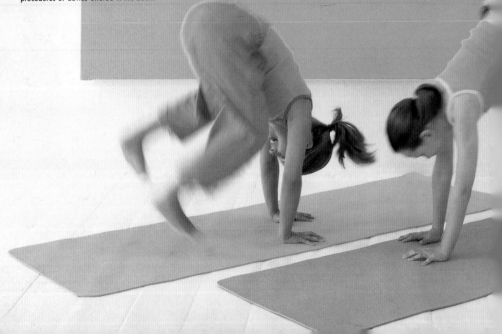

PERSONAL TRAINER
YOGA FOR KIDS

The at-home yoga class
for new beginners

LIZ LARK

Photography by Clare Park

contents

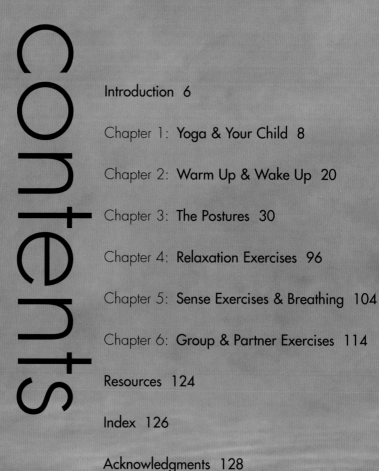

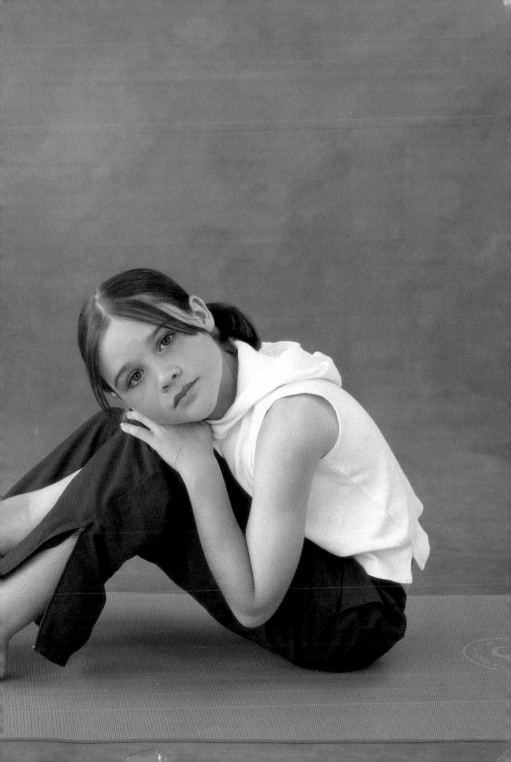

Vivid memories of kids are indelibly imprinted on my mind for ever. In 1984, while I was working during a gap year in Murree, a Himalayan hillstation school, two children called Fatima and Raazia would smile at me deliciously during break, calling 'Miss Lizzie!', with thick bread wads in one hand and hot buffalo milk in the other. Visiting them at night, they would jump inexhaustibly up and down like frogs on their thick woven *razais*, duvets made of mountain sheep's wool. For those two faces in the Pakistan Himalayas I dedicate this book, wherever they may be now, and to my nephew and niece, Ben and Philippa.

My second memory: sitting by a lake bursting with white lilies in Kodaikanal, another hillstation in Tamil Nadu, Southern India. An echo of growing laughter brought with it a bunch of wild kids on the end of huge pogo-sticks cut from trees, twice their size, arriving merrily at the lake's edge in great leaps. Here they began to plop, giggling their unbottled laughter into the water, watching me now and then. After several minutes of play and mischievously pointed nods, they drew closer, wading through the lilies. One by one each child climbed out of the water, dragging behind them garlands of sopping wet flowers. As I watched silently, they began to lay garland upon garland of lilies, which they had threaded together in the waterbed of the lake, around my neck. Dumbstruck in wet honour by this adornment, I basked in their wide-eyed smiles as they pogoed away, left speechless by these kids who made wet joy from nature.

Steve Biddulph, in his book *The Secret of Happy Children*, tells the story of a Swiss doctor who compared two World War II orphanages in Europe. One was a Western field hospital, with ample provisions and nurse care, and the other a remote mountain village with minimal but adequate provisions, staffed by local villagers and surrounded by kids, dogs and goats. His observation was that the babies in the field hospital had everything material, but little in the way of affection, touch and stimulation, whereas those in the villages had only basic care, but masses of hugs and affection – and it was these babies who were thriving. The doctor deduced that children need three important requirements: frequent touch; movement (rocking, carrying, bouncing); and eye contact (smiling and a colourful environment).

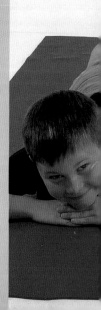

Twenty-first century kids have to contend with growing up in a crazy-paced world, tripping over itself with the stresses of busy parents and home life, coupled with raging hormones and in-your-face media and advertising. Schooling may be competitive, and it is no surprise that children become stressed, as adults do. Drawing on the techniques of yoga can empower children, as well as adults, with tools to handle stresses, moods and anxieties and can provide time-outs to cultivate self-awareness, confidence and calm amid the 'moving sea of chaos' (which yogis call *samsara*). Being the daughter of a priest, I feel a strong need to find those positive meeting points that link people of all cultures and religions, and I find that yoga provides a universal language that can help an individual deepen their personal spirituality, philosophy or sense of meaning. Essentially, yoga cultivates a childlike mind, untainted by conditioning, keeping the door to the garden of Eden open.

'When I was young, the mountains were the mountains, the river was the river, the sky was the sky. Then I lost my way, and the mountains were no longer the mountains, the river no longer the river, the sky no longer the sky. Then I attained *satori* [enlightenment], and the mountains were again the mountains, the river was again the river, the sky was again the sky.'

TRADITIONAL ZEN SAYING

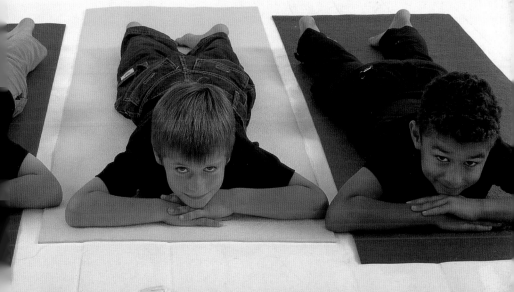

' 'TIS AN UNWEEDED GARDEN,

THAT GROWS TO SEED; THINGS

RANK AND GROSS IN NATURE

POSSESS IT MERELY.'

HAMLET

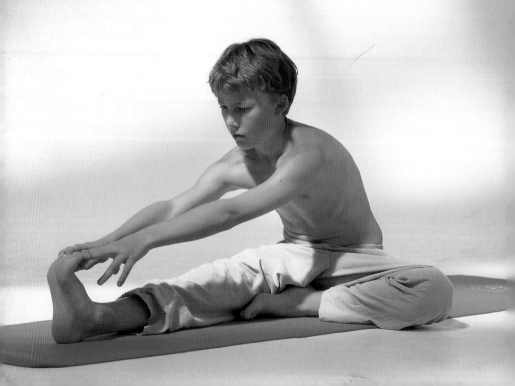

YOGA & YOUR CHILD

Children are like a canvas, absorbing paint and colours easily, and they will pick up, imitate and learn from all the influences they are exposed to, imbibing knowledge from their parents, teachers, surroundings and friends. They are amazing conduits of energy and positivity, and adults can gain much from observing their intrinsic natures. Yoga provides an ideal meeting place for mutual growth and understanding, allowing adults to grow alongside the children in their worlds.

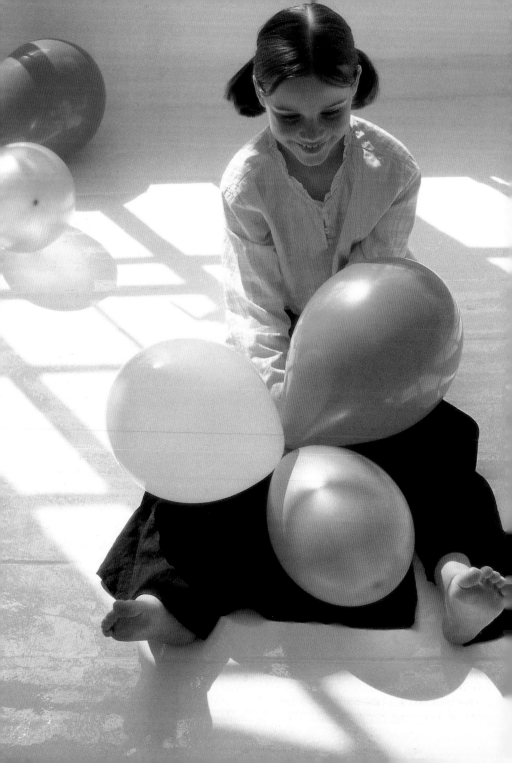

'Earth by her nourishment binds the tree,

Sky by its light keeps setting it free.'

RABINDRANATH TAGORE, BENGALI POET

THE WHOLE CHILD

It is useful to think of the body and the mind as a garden, and the seeds that are planted in the garden are sown with every impression we receive – they mould our behaviour and view of the world. Every time we are given positive, affirming messages we grow, but when negative, hurtful impressions come, we recoil. Just as a plant needs nourishing, supportive soil free from danger and poisons, and healthy external stimuli, so do we. Yoga gives us tools to empower ourselves: to clear the garden of the body of negative seeds (expressions that can become habits and what Jung called 'complexes') and learn to cultivate healthy ones, through the exercises of stretching, breathing, and positive mind-training, plus good nutrition and rest.

The Sivananda system of yoga, founded by Swami Sivananda (a spiritual seeker and doctor born in 1887), provides five tools, or main principles, we can use to take responsibility for the garden of the body and tend it well, bearing in mind that we are always a 'work in progress' throughout our lives. These are: proper exercise (postures, or *asanas*); proper breathing (*pranayama*); proper relaxation (*savasana*, and physical, mental and spiritual rest); proper diet (a fresh, colourful, natural and balanced diet – organic where possible); and positive thinking and meditation (bringing awareness to what 'is').

In *Yoga Education for Children*, Swami Satyananda outlines how children are malleable, like metal, and easily moulded. A teacher must be responsible and impart good knowledge, which will build a healthy body and mind with a positive mental attitude. Yoga is a complete art of living well, and an interdisciplinary system of teaching, combining multiple intelligences within us. In this way, it can appeal to all children and nurture them without being exclusive, drawing out creative, discerning, sensitive, bright and happy individuals. The 'whole child' can be embraced, through storytelling, colour imagery, visualization, music, language, speech pronunciation, body articulation and drama (imitating animals and nature). In the practice of yoga, important foundation values are conveyed, which concern ecology, anatomy, nutrition, the interdependence of things, a sense of the sacredness of life and care for oneself and others. These values, in turn, build confidence, self-esteem and self-expression, vital for mental and emotional health, and forming connections with others.

Yoga is invaluable for preschool children, providing the opportunity to develop a supple, healthy physical body while stimulating creative thinking and intellectual growth. The life of the child cannot be separated into the physical and the intellectual, but must be one whole, especially at an early age while children are constructing themselves.

Tuning the Brain

Like the body, the brain is an instrument that requires tuning in order to become focused, steady, enquiring and one-pointed (*eka-grata*). The right side of the brain is associated with intuitive, spatial, lateral thinking (like a big colourful paintbox) and governs the left side of the body. The left side of the brain is associated with logical, analytic, linear thinking (it will get you from A to B) and governs the right side of the body. Both sides need to have equal value. Intuitive, artistic subjects, such as art and dance, should be developed alongside maths and science in order to unite the intellectual with the intuitive. The unification of both sides of the brain enables you to relax *and* concentrate at the same time.

To help balance the right and left hemispheres of the brain, relaxation techniques such as *yoga nidra* and tratak are practised (see pages 102–3 and 106). Structured breathing (*pranayama*) and yoga sleep (*yoga nidra*) will refresh the brain, while listening techniques (inner silence, *antar mouna*) help the imagination to grow freely. The brain is a physical organ and requires more oxygen than any other part of the body, which is achieved with inverted, 'topsy-turvy' postures.

In order to learn, the physical body needs to be deeply relaxed, the breath free, the emotions stable and the mind focused. People tend to learn best in a relaxed and calm atmosphere, not a regimented one, where they can hold 'attention without tension'.

'It is little short of a miracle that modern methods of instruction have not already completely strangled the holy curiosity of enquiry, because what the delicate little plant needs most, apart from initial stimulation, is freedom; without that it is surely destroyed.'

ALBERT EINSTEIN

GUIDED PLAY, CREATIVITY AND COMMUNICATION

At preschool age, kids' imaginations are vivid, so games and guided play are ways of focusing attention and providing purposeful activity, without being regimental. The child is actively involved and learns through all the senses, which helps to cultivate Einstein's 'holy curiosity'. Repetitive exercises bring discipline and stimulate creativity, encouraging a receptive attitude towards active enquiry.

The sense and group exercises on pages 104–23 are good techniques for stimulating children's natural joy and imagination. Any of the suggestions overleaf will make your yoga session more varied and fulfilling.

- Music: Engage in singing, dancing, or playing an instrument. A drum or percussion instrument can be beaten while children change from posture to posture.
- Poetry: Speak or sing simple rhymes, poems and songs – either those you know or ones you make up. Chant a mantra for positivity, repeat a phrase to lift the spirits, or offer a thought for someone who needs support.

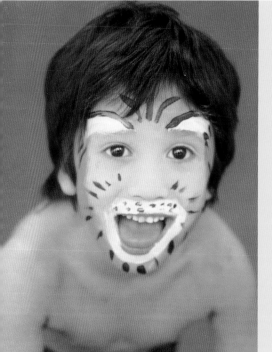

Face Painting

Try painting your face so that you really look the part. For the Lion pose, for example (see pages 56–7), first cover your face with orange face paint, then paint the centre yellow, leaving an orange rim around the edges. Use white paint around your mouth and above your eyebrows, then add on black markings and whiskers. You'll feel as brave as a lion in no time.

When designing an animal face, limit your palette to three or four colours. Draw the design on paper and colour it in first if you like. Always follow the paint manufacturer's instructions.

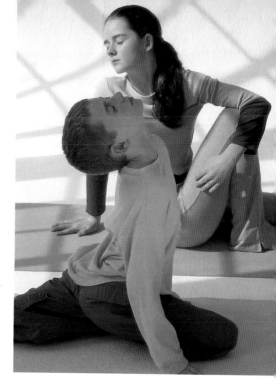

- Nature: Exploring and immersing ourselves in nature – touching the earth, squelching in mud, walking in rain – is of great value to children and adults. Kids who live in cities especially need this contact. Throughout this book we describe and copy elements of nature, such as trees, flowers and animals, and explore their qualities. Remember, too, that yoga can be practised anywhere: outside in the fresh air in a quiet spot by a tree will make the experience a beautiful one. The animal postures in Chapter 3 have been grouped into environments – sky, water, wild and earth – and pictures of these could be drawn or crafted.
- Fun: It is vital to enjoy learning and to have a purpose, but imperative to have fun along the way, too.
- Hope: Positivity is always nurtured in yoga practices, teaching and guidance. Enthusiasm is a precious commodity but it cannot be bought – children have it instinctively. Do not squash it at any cost.

Communication is essential for mental and physical health, so take time for conversation, feedback and sharing. Chris Wade, headteacher at Winns Primary School in Walthamstow, England, comments on the value of active listening: 'Children are wise. They don't have the baggage... Listen to them... What are they saying? Have a feedback (circle) time. How do they feel? Give them the language to talk to you. Ask them questions. Use simple language so they can understand.' She continues, 'Often when a child is upset, she may say, "I have a tummy ache," but what she really means is "I'm sad". Children need to be helped to express what they are feeling, to name their emotions in order to recognize and accept them, or they may express this in their behaviour. Active listening on the part of the adult is invaluable, communicating subtle ideas about feeling, so the child can understand and embrace language to express his or her feelings.' This can be explored through asking children how the postures and sense exercises feel, and what qualities they feel the pose gives them.

The best way an adult can teach a child is by practising themselves. Children will watch, and they will know if the adult is absorbed and gaining discipline, nourishment, freedom and focus through the practice.

THE BENEFITS OF YOGA FOR CHILDREN

Yoga controls and soothes emotions, removing anxiety through stretching and breathing, and enhances mental focus and physical performance. As well as improved self-esteem, the relaxation benefits help children to sleep and rest. Learning to breathe with awareness may help kids to control their anger (releasing negativity and excess energy) and can give shy ones more confidence and self-acceptance. Yoga keeps the bones healthy, strong and aligned, and the muscles around them supple, like putty or play-dough. In fact, muscles are massaged in many of the postures. Balancing poses enhance focus, equipoise, grace and concentration. They awaken creativity and fine-tune the mind. Poses named after animals and geometric angles encourage imagination and play, combined with strength, fitness and discipline. Weight is regulated and the 'whole' child is treated – mind, body, emotions and spirit.

In addition, yoga allows for freedom from religious dogma. All philosophies and religious disciplines can be embraced and deepened, though its roots are in the ancient Indian culture. Now more than ever we need to

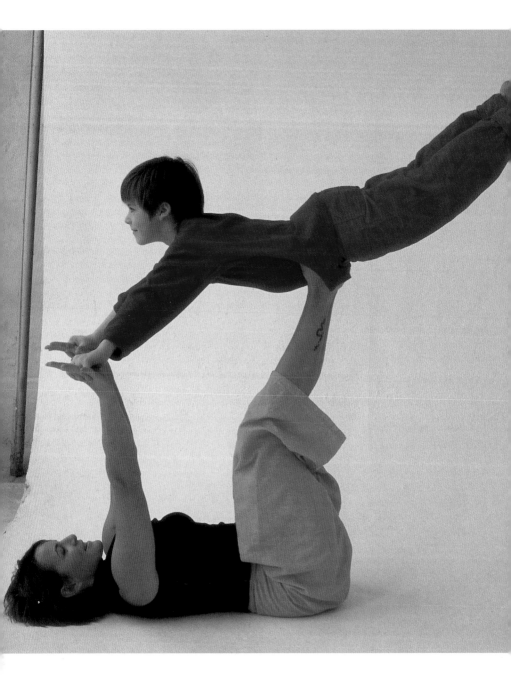

rid the world of racism, and yoga is all-inclusive and expands the mind and heart to embrace differences between peoples. Ignorance does not always mean 'not knowing' – it can mean 'wrong knowledge', which is dangerous. Yoga teaches us to stretch our minds and hearts and follow nonviolence, *ahimsa*.

Swami Satyananda, in *Yoga Education for Children*, enumerates the many direct benefits yoga can provide. Reiterated by Stacie Stukin in the *Yoga Journal*, November 2001, they include:

- Balance, stability and poise. These essential skills for sports exercise are cultivated through postures, which ensure the correct alignment of the body.
- Coordination and rhythm. As the child moves from posture to posture, these are developed.
- Concentration, discipline and focus. These increase learning faculties, develop 'attention without tension', and result in an alert, receptive and enquiring mind.
- A healthy toned body. Practising yoga will help to achieve good posture, a straight spine, supple muscles, strong bones and healthy lungs, with relaxed, free breathing.
- Flexibility and strength.
- Internal health.
- Confidence.
- Creativity and inspiration. These qualities are stimulated through visualizations, stories and guided journeys. The opportunity for self-expression leads to empowerment, which raises self-esteem.
- Courage.
- Mental health, positivity and wellbeing, including an awareness of the interconnectedness of all things, a reverence for life, and the cultivation of nonviolence, by working with one's own energies and emotions.
- Increased mental activity. This results from engaging both the mind and the body in endeavour.
- Energy and zest for life. Energy has a direct link with the structure of the spine, which acts as an electricity channel to the brain.
- Emotional and creative understanding. Exploring self-expression and practising with others develops communication skills and respect for others' ideas.
- Calmness and emotional stability.

Guna Qualities

Three qualities of nature and mind, called *gunas*, can indicate the form of yoga most useful to the child. Watch to assess which qualities are strongest in each child – *tamas* (inertia), *rajas* (dynamism) or *sattva* (illumination) – and adapt the postures accordingly. The *gunas* are always changing, and can be balanced with yoga practice.

Tamas: lethargic and slow-moving

If a child is tamasic – that is, they are indolent, have slack attention and daydream a lot – then he or she needs more stimulation. Practise dynamic yoga, such as *suryanamaskar* (Sun Salutations), to boost the system, and lots of movement and games to trigger imagination and keep them engaged.

Rajas: stimulated, fiery and dynamic

If a child is rajasic – that is, they are easily distracted or hyperactive like a jumping monkey – then the nature of yoga should be relaxing and calming, so practise such exercises as *yoga nidra* (yogic sleep). However, you may need to exhaust them first with dynamic sequences!

Sattva: balanced, ripe and fresh

If a child is sattvic, they possess concentrated attention without strain and will benefit from balancing exercises. An integrated programme of *asanas*, sense exercises and relaxation will maintain the ideal sattvic state of balance.

Try to ascertain your *guna* and that of the children before a session. To work with your natural body energies, the manual of the Satyananda school suggests a dynamic practice on Monday mornings at 8.30 am, when the energy is rajasic; a soothing, pacifying practice on Friday afternoons at 4.00 pm when the energy is tamasic; and the importance of sensing the overall atmosphere in order to give the appropriate practice.

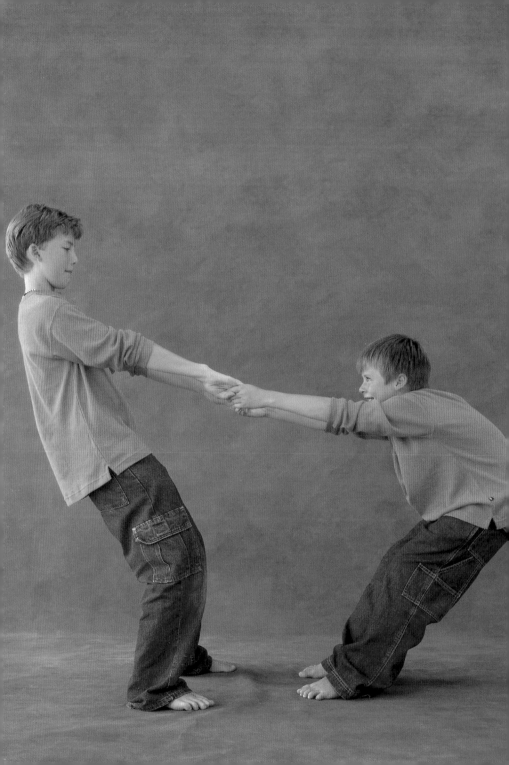

WHEN SHOULD CHILDREN START?

They can begin as early as possible, through guided play or copying adults, though structured breathing techniques should not be introduced to the under-8s. For under-8s incorporate postures and breathing exercises in games and partnerwork, interjecting appropriate exercises throughout the course of the day to help balance their energy levels (see *Gunas*, page 15). A list of yoga exercises that are only appropriate for children over the age of 8, as they require a more developed mind and body, is given on page 18.

Magic 8: The Internal Tug of War – Hormonal Haywire!

Kids grow rapidly, physically and psychologically, between the ages of 7 and 12. At 8 years old – the magic number – the lungs and immune system are developed, and children are better able to concentrate seriously. Psychologists have identified this age as that of the dawning of abstract reasoning and the understanding of concepts, morals and ideas. In India a traditional Hindu ceremony marks this time of initiation, when tensions can arise owing to the accelerated growth rate. In traditional teaching children are guided into puberty through Sun Salutations, breathing techniques (*nadi shodana* and *pranayama*) and the *gayatri* mantra, a chant important to Hindus but often also revealed through dreams to people of other cultures and traditions (i.e., because it has universal significance). From puberty the child can be introduced to all the major *asanas* and basic *pranayama*. Although meditation is not introduced until after age 21, chanting and visualizations (see pages 100–1) can be done.

When accelerated rates of physical, mental and emotional growth occur around the age of 8, fluctuating hormonal blocks can form, which can affect emotional behaviour. Glands in the body secrete hormones, which play a vital role in behaviour and mood during these adolescent years. Yoga helps to balance the hormonal system with subtle massage, especially beneficial when children are growing up so fast and hormones are going bananas! Bad moods can be soothed with yoga and yoga relaxation.

The endocrine system includes the pineal, pituitary and adrenal glands. Yogis pinpoint a significant process that happens around age 8, whereby the pineal gland, the master gland of the pituitary and the whole endocrine system, cedes its prodominant role to the pituitary gland, which releases reproductive hormones and triggers a rapid growth in emotional and mental characteristics. But this is a tragedy indeed, for the pineal gland relates to the 'third eye', the seat of intuition, which nurtures psychic and spiritual qualities and fosters emotional control. It is responsible for expanding awareness,and is devoid of sexual consciousness. The pineal gland is the 'mind's eye', the brain's control centre, linking with *ajna*, in yogic terminology, which means 'monitoring, ordering, regulating'.

We could say that until this point the child has been in the garden of Eden, balancing and discerning. The pineal is considered to be a vestigial gland that could be eventually lost for ever! However, yoga offers the fantastic possibility of nourishment to keep the 'third eye' awake. According to yogic belief, practising yoga prolongs pineal activity, leading to less aggressive behaviour and allowing a gradual emergence from the garden of Eden into puberty and sexual consciousness.

Hormones relate directly with emotions, and overactive adrenal glands (producing too much adrenaline) make a child fearful and reactive, and can lead to loss of self-control, anger and, eventually, criminal tendencies. Karma yoga (active duties, and work) as achieved in traditional ashram (a spiritual community) life, provides a useful channel for anger. An interesting story about a Buddhist *vipassana* retreat, involving ten days of silence, tells of a martial arts expert who was nearly exploding with the silence and inactivity after a few days. To channel this immense build-up of energy, he was put to work in the garden, and completed manual chores at an incredible pace!

Although living this way is not a possibility for all of us, yoga practice can combat an excess flow of adrenaline, and balance can be restored through yogic sleep (deep, guided relaxation) and alternate-nostril breathing (*nadi shodana*, see pages 110–1). Breathing and gestures (*mudras*) also soothe the nerve and glandular systems, thus reducing aggression.

Practices for Over-8s

- Dynamic postures and exercises, such as Sun Salutations and sequences of poses.
- *Shambhavi mudra*, which involves focusing or on the centre of the forehead between the eyebrows, combined with visualization. Concentrating on the forehead helps to balance mental, physical, emotional and sexual development.
- Alternate-nostril breathing (*nadi shodana*, see pages 110–11) induces calm, soothes nerves, and maintains the health and balance of the pineal gland.
- Yoga sleep (*yoga nidra*) and listening exercises (*antar mouna*) improve memory. Rotating guided journeys and visualizations (see pages 100–1) while in relaxation tap into the child's inner world.
- Mantras are soothing, deep-level sounds, which relax the brain and improve memory. It is beneficial to sing in different languages – sing mantras (sound phrases) or kirtans (simple spiritual songs) to help connect with the subconscious and calm the mind.
- Yantra breathing is a sense exercise (see page 113) that combines breathing and concentrating on a visual source, such as a geometric design, the shape or shade of a flower, or numbers on a blackboard written in different colours of chalk.
- Visualization exercises. Children who start yoga early are able to see a word, visualize it, and memorize it by making a picture in the 'mind's eye'. This skill can facilitate spelling, reading and other subjects.

GETTING STARTED

Before you begin a yoga session with children, run through the checklist, opposite. Start by examining the environment in which you will practise. The space should be clear of furniture, with no sharp or dangerous objects lying around, and clean. It should have a comfortable temperature, and be well-ventilated with fresh air so it is not stuffy, but without draughts. Screen each child for health fitness. Ask about surgery or injuries they have had, and check for obesity, anxiety, or any factor that may affect their ability to do the exercises.

Gauge the group individually throughout each exercise so that it can evolve organically to suit individual needs.

Because the mechanism for balance develops slowly in children, good training without force can be cultivated through one-leg balance poses, such as the Tree (see page 29). Practise and teach yoga with *metta* (loving kindness) and *ahimsa* (nonviolence). There is no perfect posture, just what each child can do to their best, without overstraining or competing.

Session Checklist

- Make sure that the space is clear of obstacles and at a comfortable temperature.
- The floor should be firm and even. Use mats or thick blankets to avoid hard landings, slipping or pressure on the body, especially in vulnerable poses like the Shoulderstand.
- Wear loose and comfortable, nonrestricting, clothes that are made of natural fibres, if possible.
- Practise yoga on an empty stomach, waiting at least two hours after eating, and drink water afterwards. However, do make sure that children are not hungry or tired before beginning.
- Preferably adults should shower before and after a yoga session, or at least wash their hands and face, as a physical and spiritual cleansing exercise. A simple hand- and face-washing for children is fine.
- Have variety, imagination, stories and fun in every practice. A story that relates to a posture can be read by a child or the adult to stimulate imagination.
- Adapt the session to suit the energy level of the children (see *Gunas*, page 15).
- Always warm up first (see limbers, pages 20–9).
- Do not introduce *pranayama* (structured breathing exercises) to children under 8 years of age, as their lungs are still developing. Instead use playful breathing techniques, as suggested on pages 108–9.

Tips to Remember

- Think of the spine as a vertical column.
- Make sure that you breathe freely.
- A practice is a framework for exploration. It is organic, always changing, just as we are, so bring it to life!
- Dynamic exercises are fantastic for kids, keeping them engaged, but do not be afraid to encourage stillness. Kids love *savanasana* (Corpse pose)!

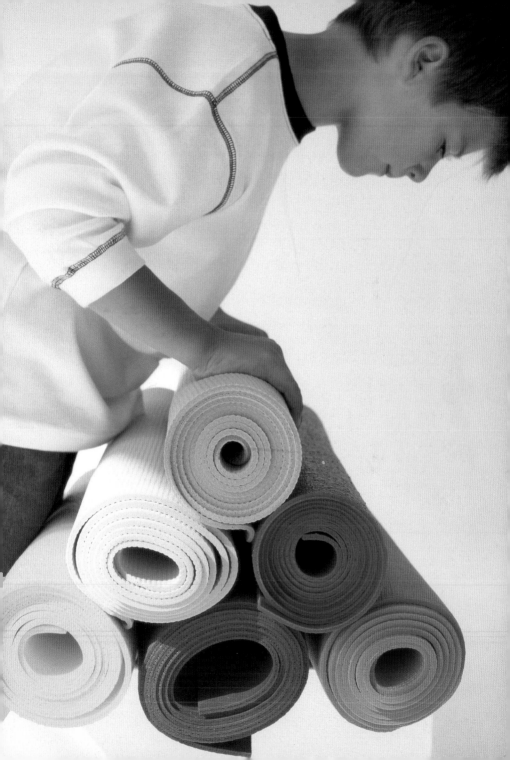

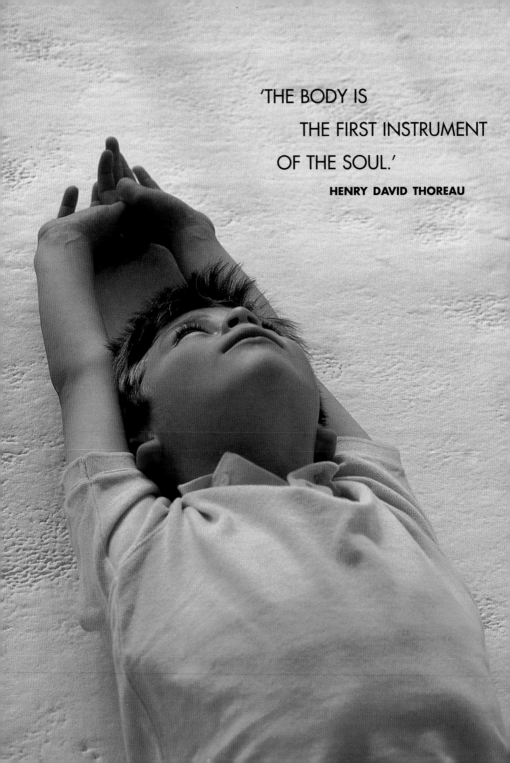

'THE BODY IS
THE FIRST INSTRUMENT
OF THE SOUL.'

HENRY DAVID THOREAU

WARM UP & WAKE UP

This chapter opens with poses to relax you and to prepare you for tuning-in to your body's alignment and breathing. The stretching 'limbers' allow you to warm up safely and fine-tune the instrument of the body in readiness to metamorphose into the postures in Chapter 3. Once you have learned these warm-ups, you will be able to use them whenever you feel angry, sad or out of sorts. By taking time out for a few minutes, you will feel happier and calmer.

CORPSE POSE

SAVASANA

This is our resting posture, very still, without exerting effort, simply breathing. Children tend to be much better at 'playing dead' like this than adults!

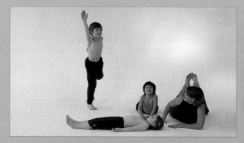

Lie face-up on the floor, with eyes closed, arms by your sides and palms facing up, and toes falling outwards. Be completely relaxed, so that if a leg or an arm is lifted, it will drop like spaghetti. Feel your tummy rise as you inhale, and fall as you exhale.

By lying as still as you can, the mind can settle into itself, rather than running off into the future or falling back into the past. Allow yourself to rest in the present moment. A few minutes in the pose is revitalizing.

HIDE-AND-SEEK WITH BREATH

Here we find the invisible breath in the body. By placing hands on three parts of the torso, we can direct the breath into each area for a three-part yoga breath.

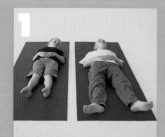

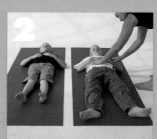

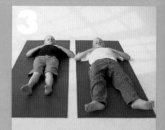

Place your hands on your tummy below your bellybutton, and take three deep breaths. Feel the movement of the breath.

Place your hands higher, cupping the ribcage, so your middle fingers touch in the centre. Take three breaths, feeling your fingers touch then part.

Now place your hands across your collarbones. Can you feel your chest lifting? It is as if you are filling a bottle with a vital drink, the breath.

PAVANMUKTASANA
WIND-RELIEVING LEG RAISES

This stretch helps balance the left and right sides of the brain, massages the tummy, eliminates excess wind and helps develop concentration, relaxation and attention.

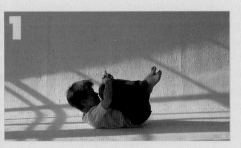 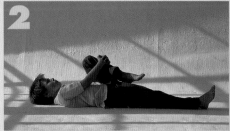

Lie on your back and curl up, clasping your knees to your chest and tucking in your head. This is called Hedgehog. Hold for five breaths, then lower your head and legs.

Clasp your left leg into your stomach, stretching your right leg out straight. Squeeze your left thigh into your tummy for five breaths. Change legs. Repeat three times on each side.

BADDHA KONASANA
BUTTERFLY

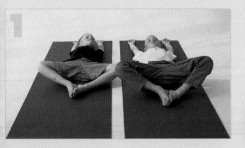 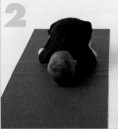 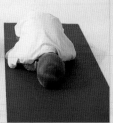

Lie on your back and drop your knees apart, with the soles of your feet touching. Stretch your arms over your head. Breathe five breaths in the lying-down butterfly pose. Flutter your wings (legs) to loosen your hips.

Curl up into a Hedgehog, as tight as you can, with your eyes closed (see Wind-Relieving Leg Raises, step 1, above). Then roll over into the Dormouse pose (see page 80), with your head tucked into your knees, for five deep breaths.

WHOLE-BODY WARM-UP

Starting from a comfortable sitting position, we will move through different body parts, warming them up one by one. We begin with the torso and head, then move on to the limbs, focusing on the shoulders, neck, face, hands and feet, squeezing and stretching these muscles to bring energy and stress-relief. Often we hold a great deal of tension in the neck and shoulders, in particular, and neck and shoulder rolls will help to keep mobility and freedom in these muscles and joints.

BENEFITS:

This all-over warm-up provides a safe, playful preparation for the more demanding asanas, bringing focus to the smaller muscles in the body and encouraging fresh blood to flow to the extremities and sense organs. The warm-up will also help to maintain flexibility and prevent the body from harbouring tensions or bad postural habits, which can lead to poor structural alignment (posture) and imbalance.

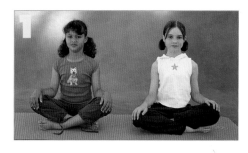

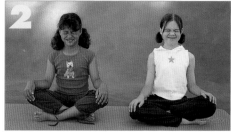

Sit on your mat with your legs crossed and your back straight. Roll your shoulders in big circles up to touch your ears, and then as far down from your ears as you can. Repeat three times each way.

Screw up your face as tight as you can, like a wrinkly prune, and say 'eeeeeeeee'. Then spread out your face as much as possible, make a big 'o' with your mouth and say 'ooooooo'.

3

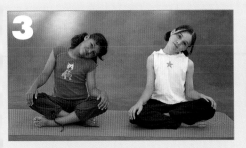

For a head roll, drop your right ear to your right shoulder, then drop your left ear to your left shoulder. Move smoothly and try not to hunch your shoulders. Repeat three times.

4

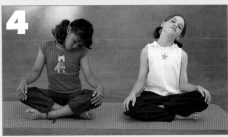

Draw a semi-circle with your head, from right ear to right shoulder, chin to chest, and left ear to left shoulder. Repeat three times in each direction.

5

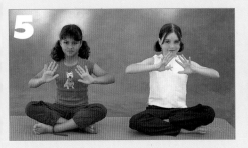

Raise your arms, bending them at the elbows and circle your hands around your wrists by flexing, pointing and rotating. Repeat three times in each direction.

6

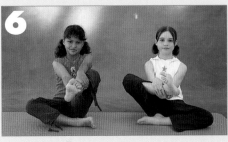

In the same way, but clasping the ankle to give support, circle your foot around an ankle, one way and then the other. Repeat three times in each direction for both feet.

7

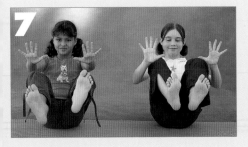

Now, raising your feet off the floor, spread your toes and fingers open as wide as you can, as if they are yawning! Coordinate the stretch in your feet and in your hands so you spread out every single toe and finger.

8

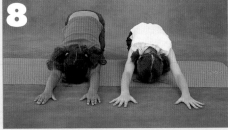

Finally, kneel and drop your head to the floor, with your arms extended, for five deep breaths. This is a Raised Dormouse, also known as the Child's pose (see pages 80–1). It is a good posture to rest in if you become tired.

SURYANAMASKAR

WAKE UP TO THE SUN

This balancing sequence stretches and disciplines the body through repetition. There are many different variations of Sun Salutations, but here the dynamic jumping variation has been chosen to help you wake up to the day with energy and focus. Repeat the 10-step cycle three times to wake up your body and get the blood circulating, so you feel alive and bright for the start of your day.

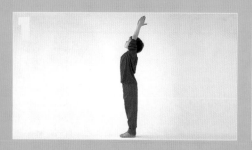

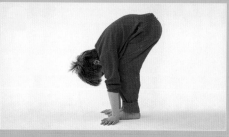

Stand in Mountain (see page 28), but with feet together and hands at sides. On inhale reach up to the sky in a wide circle, looking up, with your arms like an arrow.

Exhale, folding your body into a forward bend (see Ragdoll, page 36), dropping your head down to your knees and touching the floor with your hands.

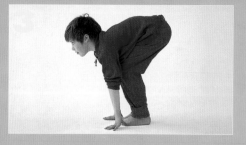

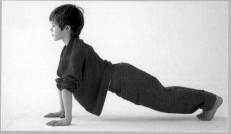

Inhale, look up and stretch out the tummy wall, lifting your chest forwards but keeping your fingers on the floor. Keep your arms and legs as straight as you can and continue looking forwards.

Exhale, spring your legs back and lower your body down to hover just above the floor, elbows bending into the sides of your ribcage, supporting your weight on your hands, the balls of your feet and the toes.

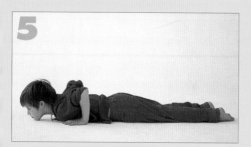

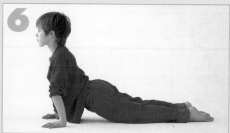

Lower your body to the floor, with elbows bent, and rest your chin on the floor (if you find it difficult to hold your weight in step 4, just lie in this position).

Inhale, look up, arch your spine and lift off the floor. Open out the chest area by drawing back the shoulders, feeling the stretch across the collarbones. Take five deep breaths.

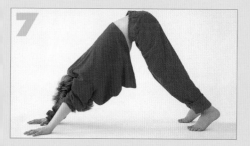

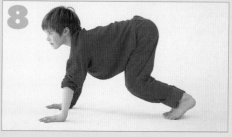

Exhale, tuck your toes under and lift your hips up to the sky, making a mountain or tent shape. Breathe five deep breaths, stretching out the back of your body.

Get ready to spring your legs forward to change into a standing bend position. On inhale, bend your knees, look up, and...

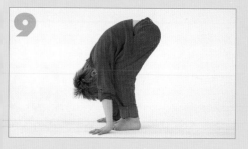

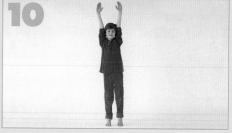

Jump your feet back between your hands. As you exhale, fold your head into your legs in a deep standing forward bend. Try to keep your legs as straight as possible and your hands on the floor. Take five deep breaths.

Inhale and draw a wide circle with your arms as you reach up to a Raised Mountain (see Puppet, page 36). Look up to the sky. Exhale, bringing your arms to your sides and standing in Mountain pose once more.

WAKE UP TO NATURE

Different postures can be combined in a linked sequence to energize and cleanse the body, like sending a positive charge through your body. In this sequence of standing postures, which includes Mountain and Tree variations, hand gestures (called *mudras*) bring detail and focus to the exercise. The Tree posture gives the feeling of being rooted firmly in the earth and being able to survive on your own. Becoming a tree feels like entering a place of trust and stability, while reaching out. All balancing postures combine this feeling of 'taking root to fly'. You may like to try making up your own sequence from the postures throughout the book.

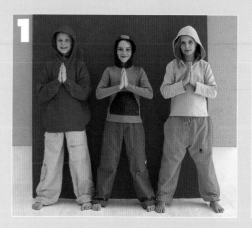

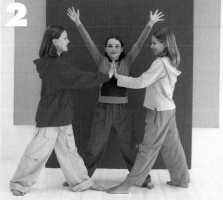

Stand with your legs 90 cm (3 ft) apart and face forwards, making sure that the spine is straight and long like a plant stem and the crown of the head is lifted towards the sky. Place your hands at the centre of your chest in the prayer position, called *namaste*, which is the universal peace *mudra*. Keeping tall and straight like a mountain, take five deep breaths to focus. This is Mountain pose.

Now inhale and reach your arms overhead like the branches of a tree, stretching your palms and fingers out to the sky. Keep your feet firmly planted in the same place, like the roots of a tree.

If you are working in a group, like the children shown here, one person could make the outstretched tree shape while the others form a pattern around the tree.

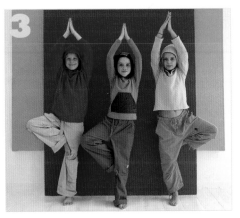

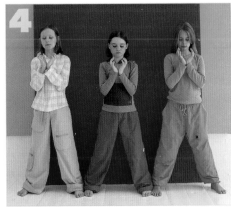

Now transform into the Tree pose. Lift your right foot with your right hand and, bending the knee to the side, plant your foot high on your inner thigh. Stand rooted into the left foot and stretch your arms up like an arrow. Look ahead and breathe for eight breaths. Repeat on the other side.

Return to the Mountain pose, and then cup your hands into the Lotus-flower *mudra* (see page 85). Open the petals and look down into the cup of your hands. Take a few deep breaths, visualizing the flowerbud opening at its heart. Gather your wishes and put them in.

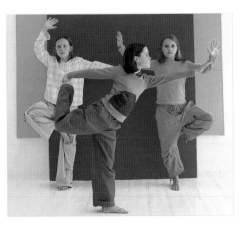

BENEFITS:

Balancing postures develop focus, harmony, poise and concentration. Mudras calm the mind and help you turn inwards.

BALANCING VARIATIONS

Now explore different ways of balancing on one leg, moving your arms, legs, torso and head in various directions, reaching, stretching, clasping and letting go. Once you have settled into a balancing pose, hold your gaze on one still point, called *drishti*, which will help you to balance and to focus your mind and body.

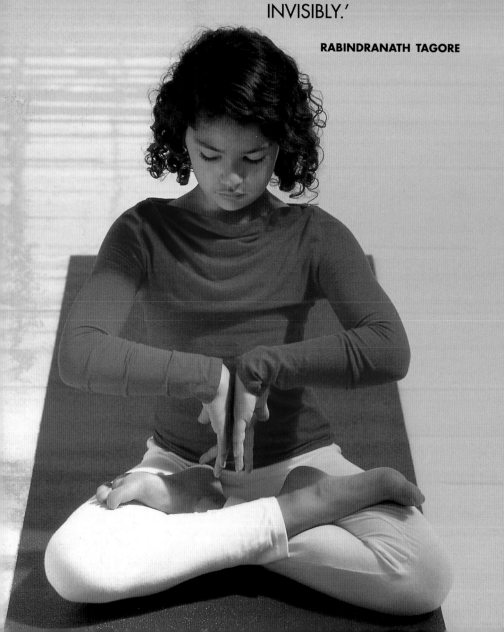

'THE JASMINE BUD IS NOT AFRAID TO BE TINY; FULLNESS REIGNS IN ITS HEART, INVISIBLY.'

RABINDRANATH TAGORE

THE POSTURES

Each animal pose in this chapter has a short introduction, which can be read by the adult or a child, and which aims to fire the imagination and encourage real involvement in each pose. Rather like Lewis Carroll's dream-child Alice, who, 'moving through a land of wonders wild and new/In friendly chat with bird or beast – half-believes it true', an imaginative child will enjoy the fantasy, and their yoga experience will be more relaxed as a result.

TRIANGLE INTO HALF-MOON

The Triangle and the Half-Moon create beautiful angles in the body and help to develop strong skeletal and muscular alignment, and enhance body carriage.

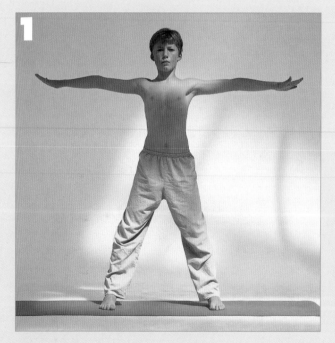

BENEFITS:
Both postures strengthen the legs, develop balance and poise, and will bring harmony, courage and the ability to focus well, too.

Stand with your feet 90 cm (3 ft) apart with strong, straight legs and a long spine. Stretch your arms out to the sides like aeroplane wings and imagine they are 3 m (10 ft) wide. Lengthen the back of your neck, lifting the crown of your head up to the sky.

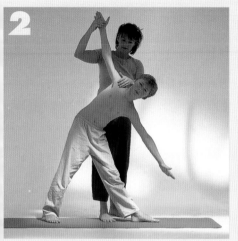

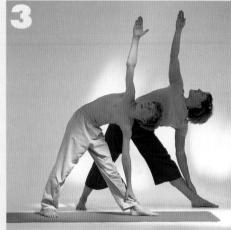

Turn the toes of your right foot inwards slightly and rotate the left foot out 90 degrees. Exhale and stretch out to the side, reaching your left arm towards the ground. Keep the chest area open, the hips facing forwards, and make sure your weight is distributed equally on both feet.

Hold on to your left leg with your left hand, and then focus on reaching the raised right arm straight upwards, as high as you can. Turn your head and look up along your arm. Open out the chest area, drawing back the shoulders, and take five deep breaths into your lungs.

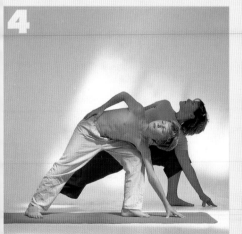

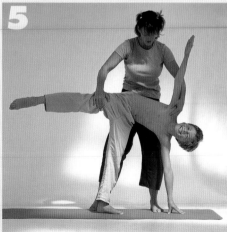

Bring your right arm to rest at your side, keep the chest area open and draw back your shoulders. Bend your left knee and place your left fingertips on the floor.

Inhaling deeply, lift your right leg firmly out to the side. Stretch your right arm to the sky. Take five deep breaths. Stand up slowly. Now repeat on the right side.

JANU SIRSASANA
HALF-BUTTERFLY

The name for the Half-Butterfly in the ancient language of Sanskrit is *janu sirsasana*, with *janu* meaning 'knee' and *sirasa* meaning 'head', so in this posture we draw the head to the knee. When you perform the pose, imagine that your right leg forms half a butterfly wing and draw it as wide as you can to warm up your hip joint and inner thigh.

There are 15,000 species of butterflies, and most of them are brightly coloured; the scales that cover them can produce iridescence – meaning that they glow with many different colours when the sun shines on them. When insects such as butterflies and fireflies go through several stages of growth before becoming adults, this is called metamorphosis, and it is similar to our human stages of development, from infant to adult. There are four stages of butterfly growth: egg, caterpillar, pupa or chrysalis, and finally the butterfly. The chrysalis is like a busy factory inside a still exterior. Some butterflies have eyespots on their wings (like the peacock's ocelli) and the peacock butterfly, with its reddish-brown wings and purple eyespot, is one stunning example. When the eyespots of the peacock butterfly flash suddenly in the light, they startle the insect's predators, giving the butterfly time to escape.

BENEFITS:
Not only does this posture stretch the lower back, and keep the hips free and flexible, it also massages the tummy on the forward bend, helping to stimulate digestion and to give you energy. It is soothing for the brain as well.

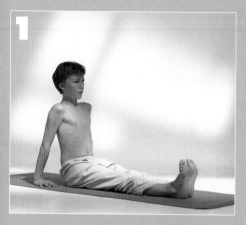

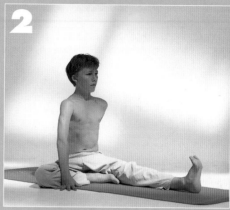

Sit with your spine straight and palms on the floor at your sides. Stretch out your legs in front of you, with feet flexed and toes spread wide like a fan. Look ahead and breathe easily. This is called the Seated Staff (see also page 41).

Now pick up your right foot and place it along the top of your inner left leg. Draw your right knee right back, as far as you can, to open out the right hip. Make sure that your chest faces directly over your straight left leg.

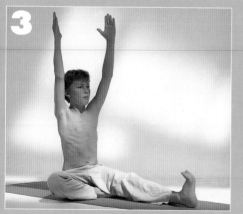

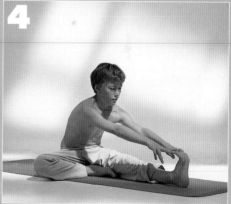

As you inhale deep into your lungs, reach your arms up over your head, pulling up through the sides of the waist and your lower back. The side of your folded right leg and the back of your left leg should remain pressed to the floor, and you should be sitting on both seat bones equally, not favouring one or the other.

As you exhale, reach forwards to catch your toes with the fingers of both hands. Do not hunch your shoulders – focus on relaxing them down and away from the ears instead. Facing your left foot, and keeping your hips square and your left leg straight, take five deep breaths. Ease out of the pose now and repeat it on the other side.

VIRABHADRASANA ▸▸

WARRIOR A

This posture suggests a powerful warrior, with tremendous strength, stability and focus. One of the main components of the yoga path is *ahimsa*, nonviolence, so this warrior is without weapons. It takes courage to dispel your fear and walk unarmed.

BENEFITS:
The Warrior posture, which is just one version of several, works to develop a strong and pain-free back. It tones and stimulates the abdomen, which is good for the internal organs.

PUPPET/RAGDOLL

This sequence incorporates a standing forward bend and the Raised Mountain pose. Practise this exercise before you move on to the Warrior, Hero and Archer.

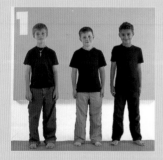

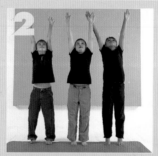

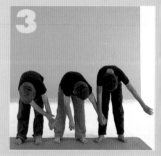

Stand facing the front, with your feet firmly planted on the floor, hip-width apart. Imagine you are a puppet. Most of the strings are slack, so relax your shoulders, but feel the one from the top of your head pulling you out of your body towards the sky.

Inhale, and reach up as high as you can, rising on to your toes – the puppeteer has picked up the strings attached to your hands. But imagine you have roots through your toes to anchor you firmly in the earth. Try to really feel this deep, two-way stretch.

Flop into a forward bend, folding your torso at the hips; you can either still be a puppet or you can turn in a ragdoll. Swing from side to side and, as you exhale, make a humming noise – think of a willow tree with a breeze moving through its leaves.

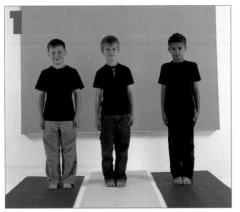

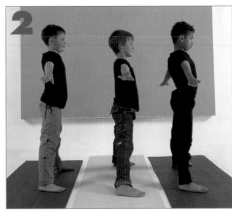

Stand tall in Mountain (see page 28). Try to keep that pulled-up 'puppet' feeling but make sure that your toes are spread, to give you strong 'roots' in the earth.

Take a deep breath and jump your feet 1.25 m (4 ft) apart. Stretch the arms out to the sides and lift your head skywards to become a five-pointed star.

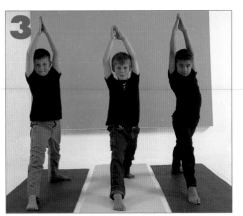

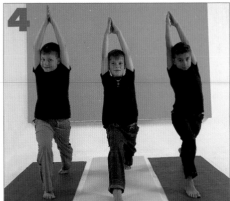

Stretch your inner legs, as if you are pulling your thighs up on to the bones. Raise your arms. Turn your left foot in, rotate both your right foot and hip through 90 degrees, and open out the chest area, broadening the collarbones.

As you exhale, bend your right leg into an angle of 90 degrees at the knee. Hold the posture, as still as you can, and breathe for five breaths. This is called Warrior A: rock-steady and focused, you are powerful.

Inhale, straighten both legs and swivel to face forwards again, slowly lowering your arms. When ready, repeat the posture, this time bending the left leg.

To finish, inhale, straighten both legs and swivel to face forwards. Then, as you exhale, jump your legs together. Return to Mountain, staying tall and brave.

HERO VIRASANA

While all other yoga postures should be practised on an empty stomach, you can go into Hero pose soon after you have eaten because, in stretching out the stomach and soothing the internal organs, it helps digestion. When you stretch backwards in this pose, you strengthen your spine so it becomes fine and lithe like a reed. You also provide a cleansing space for your abdominal organs to 'sit well', giving them space to relax and function by separating the pelvis from the ribcage. The Hero posture relaxes and opens out the chest, or heart, area. While you are doing this pose you may like to think about what qualities a hero possesses, such as fearlessness, focus, determination, discernment, dedication and passion. Other words may spring to mind as well, but always remember that a hero must have a heart for their endeavours to be worth while. He or she must choose a path with their heart, otherwise all their powerful qualities could lead to destruction.

BENEFITS:

The Hero pose is good for the joints in the legs and shoulders, and will alleviate stiffness. It helps to keep the back strong and flexible. It also stretches the feet beautifully; see how it shapes the arches of your feet so that you will have a springy step! The suptavirasana variation (see step 4, opposite) – lying down in a backbend – is especially good for strengthening the back and increasing elasticity in the lungs.

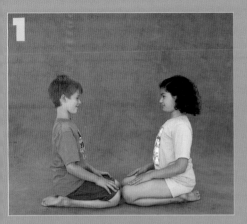

Assume the Downward Dog pose (see page 80). Then bend your knees, and sit between your ankles. This is called *virasana*, which means 'hero'. Hold for five breaths.

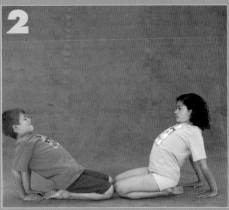

Interlock your fingers behind your back and pull them into a stretch for five breaths. Then place the hands on the floor behind you, fingers facing forwards, arms straight.

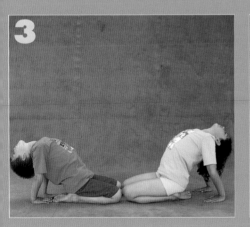

As you inhale, stretch away from the groin and arch your back, lift your collarbones and gently drop your head back. Transfer your weight to your hands and hold for five breaths.

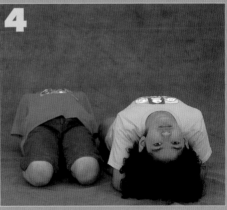

Now try to reach *suptavirasana*. Lie back in a powerful backbend, resting gently on your elbows. Lift your chest and place the crown of your head lightly on the floor.

Come out of this position very gently and then rest your lower back by curling up tightly in the Dormouse pose (see page 80). When you feel refreshed, yawn and stretch to wake up.

SANDWICH INTO ARCHER

PASCHIMOTTANASANA
AKARNA
DHANURASANA

Also called the Telephone or the Shooting Bow, this sequence starts with the *paschimottanasana*, then progresses to the seated *dandasana* and the Archer. The word *akarna* means 'to the ear' and in the pose you will bring your foot to your ear. When Buddha was about to become enlightened (meaning 'fully awake'), he sat under a bodhi tree determined to remain there until he worked out the causes of humankind's sufferings. He was tested many times by obstacles meant to throw him off balance. One test came in the form of arrows. As he sat motionless in his concentration, arrows were shot at him, directed towards his heart. He managed to sit absolutely still through this onslaught, and as soon as the arrows touched his heart they turned into lotus flowers, and fell softly to the ground around him.

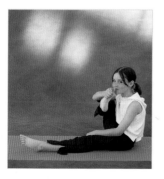

TELEPHONE VARIATION
Drawing your legs back like a bow is a little like picking up a telephone receiver. As a fun game, make a ringing sound. At the third ring, answer the telephone, taking your right foot to your ear as the receiver. Quick! The other telephone on your left side is ringing now. Next touch your toe to your nose, to your forehead, and then give your big toe a kiss! Repeat on both sides.

BENEFITS:
The Archer limbers the hips and helps to bring more flexibility to the spine and, in particular, the lower back.

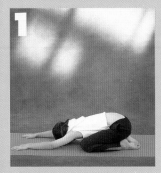

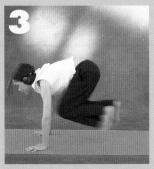

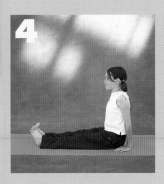

From the Dormouse (see page 80), reach your arms forwards, bringing your knees wide to open out the hips.

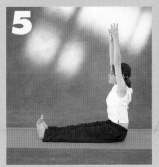

Wake up into a Downward Dog stretch (see page 80). Drop your head and push your hips to the sky.

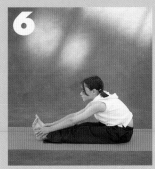

Spread your fingers. Bend the knees, look forwards, and spring your legs through your arms, to sit down.

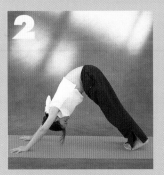

Stretch your legs out to the front. Sit with the back straight and your palms on the floor beside you. This is Seated Staff, the basic seated yoga pose (see also page 35, step 1).

Inhale, reaching the arms up over your head. Exhale and fold down to catch your toes, trying to avoid hunching or curling, in order to keep your back as straight as possible.

This is also called Tuning the West. With the feet flexed, it stretches the back (the 'west' of the body).

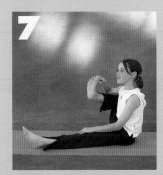

THE ARCHER

To progress from the Sandwich into the Archer pose, hook the fingers of your right hand around the big toe of your right foot; gently straighten your back, lifting your right leg and bending it at the knee; and bring your foot as close as you can to your right ear, as if preparing to fire a crossbow. Look straight ahead. Hold for five deep breaths, resting your other hand on your thigh (or using it to help draw your leg towards your ear). Now release your leg, rebalance in Seated Staff, and begin again, this time raising the left foot.

GARUDASANA EAGLE

The word *garuda* means both 'eagle' and 'king of birds' in Sanskrit. Eagles certainly are large hunting birds, and their broad wings and acute eyesight, sharp talons and hooked beaks are ideally adapted for preying on small mammals, birds or fish. Aesop's fable of the 'Eagle and the Arrow' illustrates how, even if we are strong, we can supply our enemies with the weapons of our own destruction if we are not vigilant. In the story an eagle soaring high is spotted by an archer, who draws his bow and shoots an arrow, which strikes the eagle and mortally wounds it. As the dying eagle falls, it sees one of its own feathers in the flights of the arrow. You may like to combine the Eagle with the Archer (see pages 40–1) to act out this story in your yoga session.

BENEFITS:
This difficult balancing pose makes the legs strong and flexible, and frees your shoulders. Feel how the upper back is really stretched, as if you have a broad wingspan like an eagle.

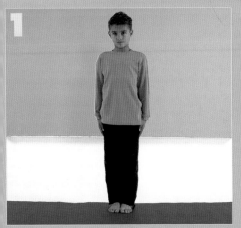

1

Standing tall in Mountain pose (see page 28), prepare for the balance by filling your mind with the great strength, quiet stealth and noble grace of the soaring eagle. When you feel ready, bend your knees a little.

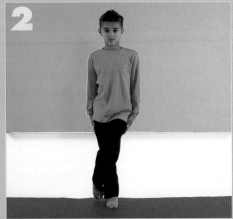

2

Shifting your weight on to your right foot, lift your left foot and wrap your left thigh over your right thigh. Try to tuck your left foot right round the back of your right calf (lower leg). Hold this balance on your right leg.

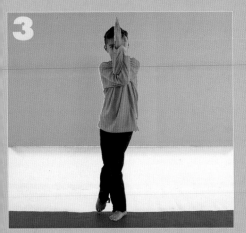

3

Now cross your right arm over your left one at the elbows, and wrap your left hand around the right, pressing the palms together. All your limbs are now woven together. Hold the balance, look straight ahead and count ten deep breaths – you must breathe, even if it is difficult to keep still. Now unwind carefully to return to standing.

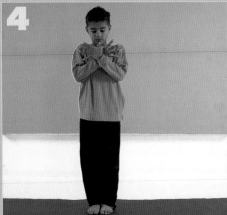

4

Mudra (Hand Gesture) Variation: If you find the balance difficult or unsettling, the *Garuda mudra* is an alternative option. Keeping your weight on both feet, cross your forearms in front of your chest with your palms facing your body. Stretch out your fingers, like wing feathers, link your thumbs together and inhale deeply for five breaths.

CRANE
BAKASANA

This balancing posture is known as the Crane. The Sanskrit word *baka* means 'crane' or 'wading bird'. When you do this pose, think of the silence and stillness of a heron fishing in the shallows, perfectly balanced, despite appearances – a disproportionately large body on stiltlike legs. It stands apparently motionless so that the fish beneath the surface are not frightened away by a moving shadow, but in fact it is poised for a dartlike attack. Similarly, contained in complete composure, the Crane posture has an abundance of energy, and in this balance you should be able to create the same potential power for yourself.

BENEFITS:
Balancing your weight on your hands will obviously strengthen the upper body and arms, but the Crane also works the tummy muscles; strong abdominals are absolutely essential if you want to be able to balance in this pose. Because trying to achieve the balance is great fun, this pose also provokes many smiles – an obvious benefit in itself!

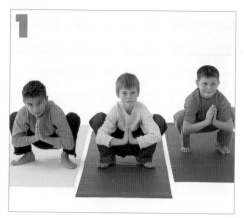

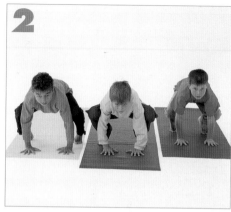

To warm up for this balance, bend your knees and assume a squatting position, looking straight ahead. You should aim to have your feet facing forwards, with your heels squarely on the floor and the soles of your feet flat. Press your hands together in the prayer position.

Place your hands firmly on the floor in front of your feet and spread out the fingers – imagine they are the crane's long toes in the river mud. Bend your elbows to make a shelf on which to rest your knees. Lean forwards and transfer most of your weight from your feet to your hands.

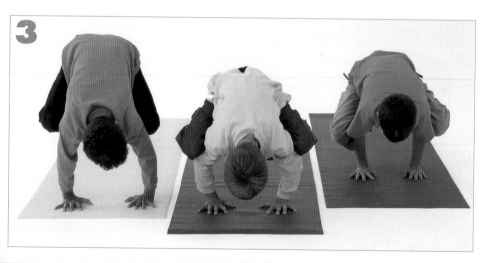

Gradually lift your heels and rise up on your toes, putting more weight on your arms and hands, before you actually try to lift your feet off the floor. When you do achieve the balance, look to the front and take five deep breaths. Then gently put your toes back on the floor.

HAMSASANA SWAN

The word *hamsa* does mean 'swan' in Sanskrit, but the real name for this posture is *eka-pada* (meaning 'one-foot') *rajakapotasana*, 'the king of pigeons', because the chest is pushed forwards like a pigeon's breast. Here I have named it the Swan because the stretch pulls through the neck. There are different ways of doing this pose, but this way creates a swan arch – a long throat with a wide, open chest. The Swan is good to do as a 'counterpose' – with a partner – if you like to make beautiful shapes. And you may like to read Hans Christian Andersen's much-loved story *The Ugly Duckling* before you begin. It will serve as a reminder that it is only by accepting what we are that we will blossom – and only if we are patient, because the growing will not necessarily be speedy. We can all emerge as beautiful swans, if we wait quietly for the white feathers to replace those stubby brown ones, rather than trying to force ourselves to be something we are not, and making ourselves unhappy in the process.

BENEFITS:
This posture allows the lungs to expand for deep breathing, making you feel brave and awake. It also tones and strengthens the spine by exercising your neck and shoulders, as well as the pelvis, the seat of the torso, and the back and upper body. What is more, the pose ends with the Raised Dormouse (see page 81), which gives a fantastic stretch to the lower back.

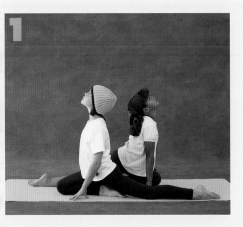

Start by kneeling down and placing your hands beside your knees with your fingertips pressed to the floor. Taking weight on to your fingers, slide your left leg backwards and straight out behind you, and tuck your right heel underneath you. Keep your toes pointed. Make sure that your right knee faces forward in a straight line with your back leg and that you are sitting on top of your right heel.

Slowly lift up your chest and head, keeping your hands – or at least your fingertips – pressed on the floor and your arms straight. Lengthen your neck in a beautiful sweeping arch and stretch your throat, breathing slowly and deeply. Look up, making sure that you keep your face very relaxed and imagine you are the queen of the swans gliding along on a silvery lake. Hold for five breaths.

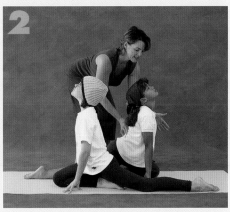

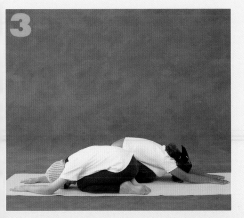

After achieving the deep back arch in the Swan posture, draw the left knee in beside the right one and curl up in Dormouse as a counterpose to soften your back and rest – the Raised Dormouse is a lovely relaxing stretch that will help to align your spine (see pages 80–1). Then repeat the Swan arching stretch and pose with the right leg extended behind you instead.

NATARAJASANA
LORD OF THE DANCE

B ecause the word *nata* means 'dancer' and *raja* means 'Lord', this posture is called the Lord of the Dance. It is best suited to older children. In Hindu culture Siva was the Lord of the Dance and of mystical stillness. He lived in Mount Kailash, a holy mountain in the Himalayas, and he is said to have manipulated his body in 840,000 ways, each representing a different bird or animal. These movements, or *asanas*, filled his body with *prana*, or 'clear energy', and allowed the god's mind to expand beyond the mundane. Many Indian sculptures in stone and bronze have been inspired by Siva's agile and graceful movements.

BENEFITS:
This pose develops balance, poise and grace, and is fairly challenging. It strengthens the leg muscles, frees the shoulders and chest, and stretches the spine in a beautiful arch.

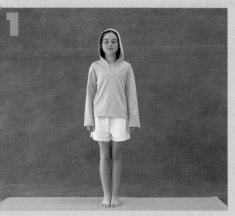

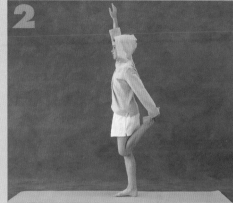

The first stage of the Lord of the Dance pose is known as the Stork. So start by standing firm and tall in Mountain pose (see page 28), and concentrate on breathing slowly and evenly. This will help to energize you for the balance to come and it will steady you, too, letting you develop strong roots in the earth beneath you.

Moving your weight onto your right leg, lift your left foot from the floor and bend your knee, to fold up your left leg behind you. Catch your foot with your left hand. Then stretch your right arm up to the sky. Look straight ahead, focusing on a fixed point, and continue to breathe steadily, keeping your face calm. This is the Stork pose.

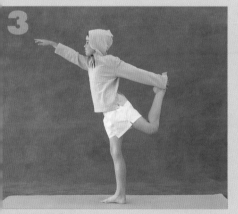

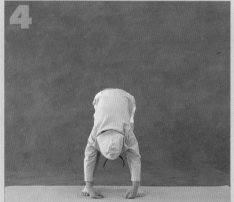

Now begin to develop the posture – by slowly leaning forwards, stretching out your right arm and raising your left leg behind you, holding it firmly with your left hand. This creates an arch similar to the one you assumed in the Swan (see pages 46–7), but here you are balancing on one leg. Lift your chest up, and take five deep breaths.

Gently release your foot and lower your left leg and right arm. Relax and flop like a Ragdoll (see page 36) for five breaths, reversing the arch to soften and rest the back. Then, in order to stretch both sides equally, repeat the balance, reaching up and out with your left arm this time and lifting your right leg. Then relax again.

MAYURASANA
PEACOCK

This pose is the first stage of the Peacock, and it uses a special hand position that strengthens the wrists. It is an advanced posture, which should really only be executed with the help of an adult, so be careful and concentrate. Practise it until you are proficient before going on to the Dancing Peacock. The male peacock is probably the most spectacularly adorned of all birds, with iridescent plumage of purple, blue-green, turquoise and gold, and many, many tail feathers which form a huge fan in display. Such exhibitionism is not an everyday event, though, and the peacock's tail generally trails heavily behind the bird, filled with jewels like the train of a coronation robe. Perhaps it might help to think of the elegance and poise of a peacock when you come to focus on this balance.

BENEFITS:
Both the Peacock and Dancing Peacock poses develop balance and poise, but especially strengthen the upper body, arms, wrists and shoulders. Eventually, as you practise, the poses will become full-arm balancing postures, like the Crane (see pages 44–5) or the Firefly (see pages 58–9).

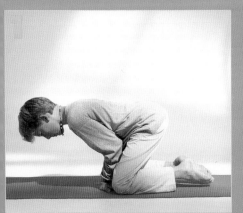

Kneel on all fours on the floor, as in the Cat pose (see pages 78–9), but then place your hands together on the floor, almost between your knees, with palms down and fingers turned back towards your body, so that the insides of your wrists point forwards. Stretch out your fingers like bird claws. You are going to balance your entire weight on your hands, so you need them to be a firm foundation.

Bend your elbows in towards your abdomen, and lean forwards, keeping the forearms together, and rising up on your knees. Rest your chest on your upper arms while the elbows press into the centre of your lower abdomen. Carefully lean your torso forwards as you balance on your hands, like a seesaw with your body (you may need to place your forehead on the mat to find your balance).

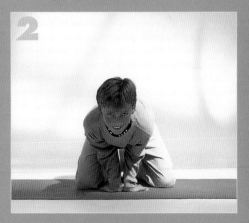

With your knees still on the floor, look forwards and imagine you have a wonderful display of bright feathers shooting up behind you in a massive fan. Smile and take five deep breaths. As you become more advanced, you might like to try – with a grown-up's assistance – to stretch out your legs behind you, so that you are holding your body in a straight line, parallel to the floor.

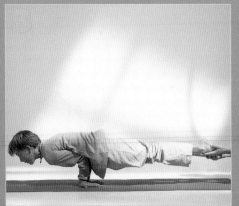

DANCING PEACOCK
PINCHA MAYURASANA

This posture is really only suitable for older children, as it is fairly advanced. Initially it requires hands-on supervision, although more proficient youngsters may like to practise it independently, using a wall behind them as a support. In Sanskrit the word *mayura* means 'peacock' and *pincha* means 'chin' or 'feather'. This spectacular elbow-balance pose mimics the peacock as it shows off its full plumage. A peacock's tail has hundreds of eyespots, called ocelli, patterns that resemble eyes, and point towards the body of the peacock. When, during the mating season, the peacock fans out its plumage and shakes its tail, the ocelli vibrate and shimmer, dazzling the female peacocks into a trancelike state. The females choose the male peacocks that have the most ocelli on their tails. Be proud of yourself when you practise this pose – like a peacock attracting attention to itself – and you will give yourself confidence. Alternatively, you could imagine yourself as a peacock in India during the rainy season, when these beautiful birds are said to dance to dry out any feathers that might get wet trailing on the ground, raising their fanlike tails again so that the wind can blow them dry!

BENEFITS:
In addition to the benefits listed on page 50, the Dancing Peacock will give you a brain-bath, supplying a fresh flow of blood to the head, and it will give your heart a rest, too.

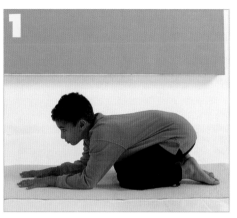

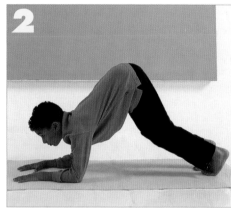

Kneel down and place your elbows and forearms square on the mat to form two parallel lines, palms on the floor in front of you. Then stretch and spread out your hands and fingers like peacock feet, your thumbs touching each other. Focus on your contact with the ground, in order to build a firm foundation for your balance.

Staying on your elbow base, lift your buttocks (tail) up towards the sky in the shape of a Downward Dog (see page 80). Keeping your head up, stretch out your legs behind you and lift your buttocks higher, resting on your toes. This is the beginning of the full Dancing Peacock posture – breathe for five to steady yourself.

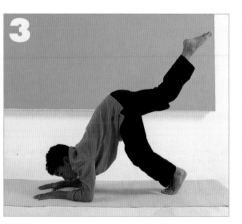

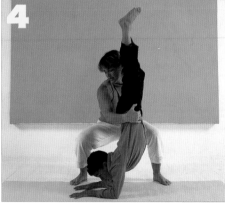

Lift the right foot off the floor, stretch your right leg up and point your toes. Hold the lift for a deep breath, then lower your leg gently, putting your weight evenly in both legs. Now repeat the balance but this time raising the left leg. Then, remembering the breath each time and lifting each leg in turn, repeat the whole sequence.

With a grown-up's help, try the full posture, but if you hurt at all, stop! Balance on your elbows, and kick up your legs one at a time so that the adult can catch them to hold you safely. Stretch up your pointed toes, legs together, and lift your shoulders away from your ears. Take three breaths, then come down into Dormouse (see page 80).

BHUJANGASANA
COBRA

S nakes are mysterious creatures – silent and sometimes deadly. They slither along with a zigzag action, pushing against objects to propel themselves forwards. They can sense their environment through their skin, and their tongues dart in and out to pick up scent in the air, telling them when food or danger is near. Snakes shed their skin between three and seven times a year, the old skin simply peeling off to reveal a brand-new one underneath. Often the old skin will be discarded in a single, snake-shaped piece. Quiet and sensitive creatures, snakes will usually hide from humans if they hear them approaching. If a snake bites you, it will probably have been in self-defence, because you were not listening and watching as you passed through its domain. In yoga we aim to make the spine feel like the spine of a snake – lithe, free, flexible and extremely strong. In this posture, which arches the spine deeply and stretches out the tummy muscles, we create a shape like a snake, as it rises up and draws its head back, about to strike its prey.

BENEFITS:
This posture heals, strengthens and aligns the spine. It opens out the chest area fully, encouraging free, deep breathing in the lungs, which feeds the blood system with fresh, oxygenated blood. The Cobra pose makes us brave because the chest is opened and lifted, so we can breathe without fear.

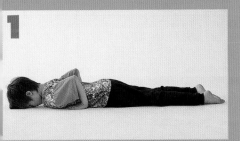

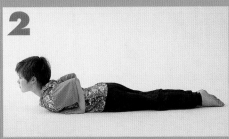

Lie face down, your forehead resting on the floor to relax your neck. Press your hands into the floor by your waist, fingers forwards. Hold your legs together and point the toes.

As you inhale, push down firmly through your hands into the floor. Think of the snake, and look up, raising your head and neck. Slowly and gently, begin to lift your torso.

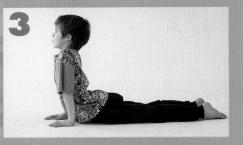

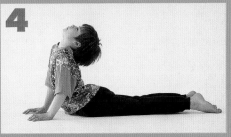

Continue the lift smoothly to raise the upper body, lifting the shoulders up and back, and finally the chest, so that your back is arched and your arms are straight.

Inhale deeply and drop your head back to arch your spine as much as you can, without straining. Feel the chest area open and your lungs lift and expand. Hold for five breaths.

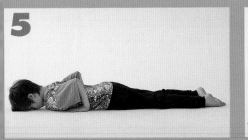

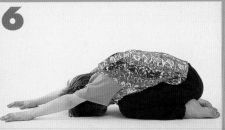

As you exhale, bend your elbows to bring your head and torso slowly out of the arch and lower yourself back on to the floor to rest. Relax for five deep breaths, with your forehead touching the floor, before you start again.

Make the arch three times, then fold your hips back on to your heels, stretch out your arms in front of you, and rest in the Dormouse or Raised Dormouse (see pages 80–1) for ten breaths. Now come up into a kneeling position.

LION SIMHASANA

In Sanskrit *simha* means 'lion', and this posture is dedicated to the lionman, named Narasimha. In the film, *The Wizard of Oz*, the Wizard was rumoured to be a terrifying hidden power, and the Lion in the story was full of fear at the prospect of meeting him, even though lions are traditionally associated with courage. The cowardly Lion was ashamed because he was supposed to have a mighty roar that would frighten people, but he seemed to have lost his ability to roar and, because of this, he lost his courage, too. But the Wizard was just as scared as the Lion, and to protect himself he hid behind huge walls and learned to shout very loudly! The truth is that he was alone and frightened, too! As the Lion in the story discovered, fear is a state of mind, and the following posture will help clear away any feelings of fear and negativity, and draw in positive energy that will help to make us feel brave and confident. This is also a good posture to try when you're feeling angry or frustrated, because it dispels tension and helps to relax you.

BENEFITS:
The Lion pose strengthens the throat and helps prevent sore throats. It also cleanses the tongue and so cures bad breath! With regular practice it brings clearer pronunciation so that speech improves. It also releases tension and rejuvenates the muscles in the face, hands and wrists.

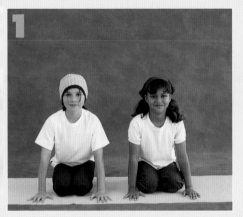

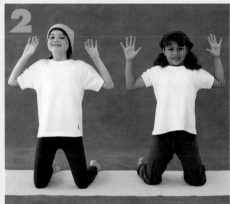

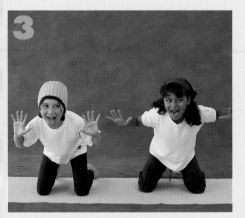

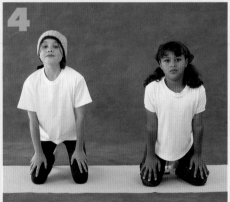

To prepare for the pose, kneel on your mat, resting your hands on your knees, and straighten your spine, lifting the chest. Then lean the trunk of your body forwards, making sure that you keep your spine as straight as possible, and place your hands on the floor, beside the knees. Think about the strength of the great king of beasts.

Then, as you inhale, grow taller by coming up strongly into a raised kneeling position. Lift your hands head-high and hold them shoulder-width apart, and then spread your fingers, like claws, to become a rampant lion. Keep pulled up at the knees and be careful not to collapse forwards at the hips, letting go of your lower back.

As you exhale, lean forwards from the hips, open your mouth wide as if to let out a mighty roar, and try to touch your chin with your tongue. Stretch your fingertips at the same time, as if you are flexing your claws. Stay in this strong position for a few moments, until you have emptied your lungs of as much air as possible.

Now put your tongue back in your mouth and relax your face, arms and hands. Lower to a kneeling position and place your palms back on your knees, so that you have returned to your starting position. Take five breaths and then repeat the posture four times, trying to grow a little – becoming more and more mighty – each time.

TITTIBHASANA
FIREFLY

The word *tittibhasana* refers to an insect, like a firefly or glowbug, that glimmers at night. It is magical to be in a forest at night with fireflies (also called lightning bugs) silently glowing among the trees, like natural fairylights. Why do fireflies light up? It is the girls' way to attract the boys, basically! Special light cells, called photocytes, on the wingless female's lower belly flash intermittently to broadcast her position. The chemicals in these cells are called luciferin and luciferase, meaning 'bearer of light', as does Lucifer, the fallen angel: in Latin *lux* means 'light' and *ferre* means 'to bear'.

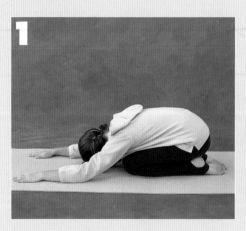

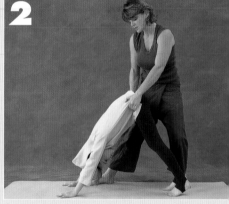

Start quietly in the Dormouse pose (see pages 80–1). It may help you to run through the life cycle of the insect in your mind – from the glow worm to the mature firefly – so that you, too, can develop gradually, stretching your wings only after a relatively still and mentally composed pupal stage (see also Half-Butterfly, page 34).

Now stretch up into a Downward Dog pose (see page 80), lifting up through your toes to stand squarely on the soles your feet, and pushing the hips up towards the sky. Open up your shoulders, and breathe steadily and deeply to prepare yourself for the balance to come. When you are calm and focused, get ready to jump!

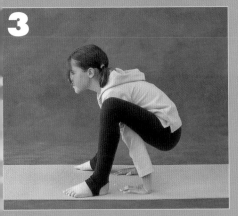

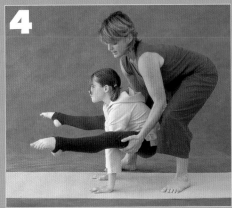

Let your energy escape in a bunny hop or leap-frog to jump your legs around your shoulders, so that your feet land outside, or in front of, your hands in a wide squat. Looking straight ahead, try to balance the thighs on your outside upper arms. Then nudge your shoulders gently through your legs so that your legs squeeze your shoulders.

Now – and you will probably need an adult's help at this point – straighten your legs wide in front of you, pull up the leg muscles, point your toes, and balance on your hands for five breaths. Lift your toes as high as possible, to drop the base of the spine towards the floor, lowering your centre of gravity and making the balance easier.

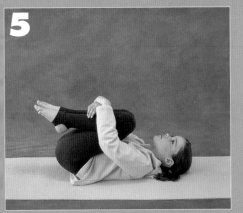

BENEFITS:
The Firefly and other arm balances develop upper-body strength. In this pose the abdomen is massaged and cleansed, and the spine is stretched in a deep forward bend. Learning to transfer weight on to your hands is challenging and exciting, but it is also fun, and having fun is always good for you!

To come out of the posture, you should lower your feet slowly to the floor and then lie on your back, curling up into a Hedgehog (see page 23). Take ten deep, refreshing breaths. Do not worry if you cannot hold the balance for long – if at all. Play with the posture, and with practise, and if you keep breathing and focus, it will improve.

CAMEL USTRASANA

Camels live in deserts – dry, barren, wild places where few animals and plants can survive. They are perfectly adapted to the severe conditions of their natural environment; their humps act as storecupboards for fat reserves, they can close their nostrils to keep out blustering sand and their huge, wide, flat feet are ideal for walking great distances in the sand. They can also drink vast amounts of water and then go for days without drinking, drawing on the reservoirs they have taken in. Although they have become man's beasts of burden, these graceful 'ships of the desert' still evoke feelings of pride and strength, and a certain mysticism. In the Sinai Desert there is a famous mountain that, if you are physically fit, you can climb by night in order to see the sun rise from the top – and what a wonderful place it is to meditate! It is a three-hour trek, with tea and a blanket at the end as reward, but if you get tired along the way you can choose to pay a few pennies to ride high upon a camel to the top. This is a truly magical experience, under the midnight-blue sky sprinkled with tiny bright stars, and with the sounds of the camel's jangling jewellery.

BENEFITS:
This keeps your back open, straight and free, and this will promote good posture, so that you can avoid getting hunched in later life. It will keep your shoulders broad and your chest free, and it stretches and massages the abdomen, too.

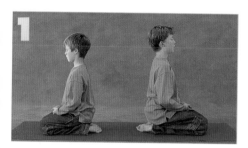

Assume a kneeling position on your mat, with your hands resting in your lap and your feet tucked under behind you. Take three deep breaths to relax and focus.

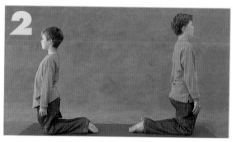

Then lift up your hips so you are 'standing' tall and straight on your knees, looking ahead. Relax your arms down by your sides and breathe deeply for three breaths again.

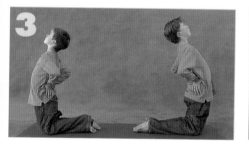

Lift your chest upwards to the sky. Rest your hands on your lower back, with the fingers pointing down. Draw your elbows back as far as you can without straining.

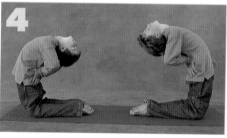

Keeping your lower legs pressed to the floor, push your hips forwards, and really arch your back, drawing your shoulders back and lifting the chest skywards.

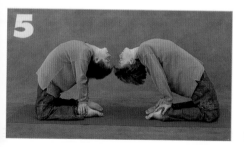

Arching your back a little more, drop your hands back to touch your feet, keeping your arms straight. Think of lifting the chest. Hold the pose for ten deep breaths, then gently let your head drop back to open out your throat.

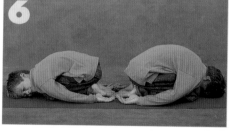

Lift up your chin gently, until it touches your chest, and then, with your hands to support your back, lift up out of the arch. Curl up into a tiny Dormouse (see page 80) to rest your back. Breathe slowly, as quietly as you can.

SALABHASANA ▶▶
LOCUST

This posture is similar to the Crocodile (see page 72), but the hand positions are different. Locusts are migratory grasshoppers, which means they fly to avoid harsh weather, to find water or to nest. Sometimes they fly in massive swarms, so big that they block out the sun, and they have destroyed whole crops by eating them.

PARACHUTING SPIDER

This Spider pose, as if you have sky-dived out of an aeroplane, is added for fun. The spider, busy spinning its web, is a good example from nature of karma yoga, where immersion in work with concentration and focus is a yoga in itself.

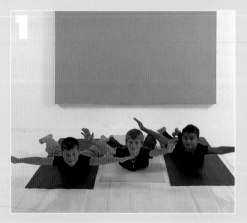

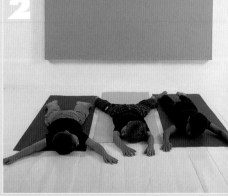

Stretch out, face down, on the floor. Take a deep inhale, and on the exhale stretch out your arms and legs as wide as you can, while lifting your head, upper torso and thighs to balance on your bellybutton.

Hold for five breaths if you can, pretending you are flying through the air, after working hard to weave your silvery web. Then lower your body, stretch out, relax and smile, enjoying the feeling of release.

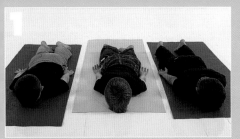

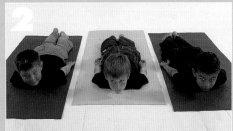

Lie very straight, face downwards, with your hands by your sides and palms facing up. Imagine you are a chrysalis, a creature sleeping in a woven womb before it hatches into a beautiful adult bug. Remain in this 'sleeping state', breathing for five breaths.

As you wake up, breathe in, lift your chin off the floor and look forwards, as you did in the Cobra (see pages 54–5), making your body very stiff, but keeping your arms by your sides. Stretching your legs, point your toes away from you, like the locust's tail.

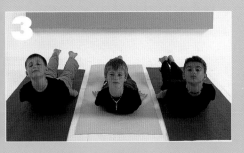

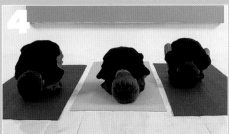

Now raise your straight legs and lift your chest, drawing back your shoulders to make your body like a stiff bow; do not bend your knees. Press your hands down on the floor and breathe in the posture for five deep breaths. Exhale, and relax to the floor. Repeat the lift three times.

As an extension of the exercise, repeat the Parachuting Spider exercise (see opposite), with your arms and legs outstretched and breathing deeply into the lungs. To counterpose, curl up into a Dormouse (see page 80); this will rest and relax your spine.

BENEFITS:

The Locust is a wonderful massage for the intestines, helping digestion and relieving constipation. Like the Cobra posture, it works on strengthening the upper torso, but here the legs are also brought into play. This is a great counterpose to Shoulderstand (see pages 92–3) because it exercises both the back muscles and the abdomen.

THE BEAR

Bears live in cool, northern parts of the world. They have large heads, thick shaggy coats and no tails, with short back legs and powerful front legs with sharp claws. They cannot see or hear well, but their sense of smell is acute. Many bears hibernate (go into a kind of deep sleep) throughout the winter. Arctic polar bears roll on icy ground to dry their thick, creamy fur after swimming, and you may find the following poem inspires you to create your own bear games and positions:

'Roly poly polar bears, rolling in the snow
Sliding over icebergs, in the sea they go ...
Growly brown mountain bears, climbing on all fours.
Hugging each other with their big, brown paws.'

CELIA WARREN

There is another bear we all know, and his name is Pooh. He is an endearing bear who thinks a lot about nothingness, as illustrated in Pooh's poem, 'Lines Written by a Bear with a Very Small Brain', by A. A. Milne. You may like to read parts of *Winnie the Pooh* before attempting the pose, to get you thinking about bears.

BENEFITS:
The Bear is a 'play' pose, and not a classical yoga posture as such. The benefits are the same as for Downward Dog, but because it involves walking, it exercises the shoulders and hips. It is also fun, which is very important for a happy, healthy heart!

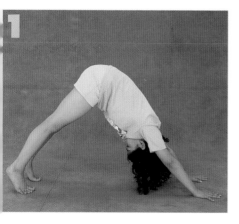

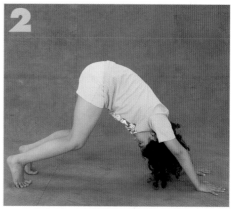

You will start the Bear from the Downward Dog posture (see page 80). From a kneeling-on-all-fours, or 'table', position, rise up on to your toes and lift your hips high up to the sky. Straighten your legs, stretch out your back, and make the spine long and lean, allowing your head to drop down between your arms.

Take five deep breaths. Bend your knees. An adult can now recite the bear rhyme opposite, and you can decide whether you want to be a white polar bear or a brown grizzly. Think about your habitat and what you will find there – an icy snow-capped world where you dive for fish, or a forest full of berries and roots to eat.

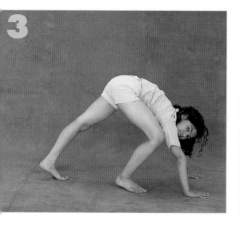

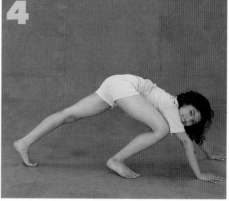

Begin to walk around the room, as if you are looking for food to eat. Walk your left hand and your right foot forwards at the same time, then your right hand and your left foot forwards. Think about the heaviness of a bear's body; keep your hips high, your limbs long and try to place as much weight on your hands as on your feet.

Smell the air to pick up any scents around you. Make the sounds of a murmuring bear, 'mmmmmmmm'. You are a contented bear. Hum a tune. As you hum, begin to move faster into a bear gallop, moving as smoothly and rhythmically as you can. Remember that bears cannot see or hear very well, but can smell everything around them.

URDHVA CRAB DHANURASANA

The Crab pose is not for beginners and it requires an adult's guidance, as it is a powerful, exhilarating backbend. The word *urdhva* means 'upwards' and *dhanu* means 'bow' in Sanskrit, and in the pose a deep arch, or bridge, is created that stretches the body into a beautiful arching bow, like an instrument, finely tuning the spine. In fact, the pose is usually called the Upward Bow by yoga practitioners, but here I am calling it the Crab because the shape is like the arch of a crab shell, and the hands and feet can walk as a crab does, sideways.

Crabs are crustaceans – they have a shell-house. There are so many different kinds, with such descriptive names as hairy crab, slender-legged spider crab and sponge crab, but the one I like best is the hermit crab. This one has no hard shell to protect it, so it lives in other, empty, shells. It is like a wandering *sannyassin* (spiritual seeker), and can be found in rock pools, growing to about 10 centimetres (4 inches). Look out for a hermit crab on your next trip to the beach!

BENEFITS:
A beautiful posture, the Crab maintains life and vitality in the spine, and will strengthen the arms, wrists, legs and ankles. Like all the other backbends, it also keeps the heart, or chest, area open, thus encouraging emotional freedom and open expression.

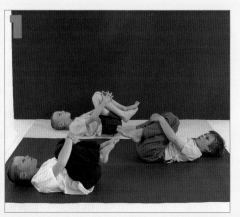

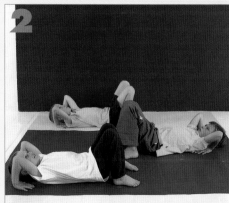

Lie on your back and curl up into a tiny Hedgehog (see page 23), clasping your knees to your chest but without tucking in your head. Pull your knees tight into your chest to stretch out your spine for five deep breaths, and then release them slightly. You may like to rock back and forth gently to warm up your spine even more.

Now uncurl and place your feet on the floor close to your buttocks, with the knees pointed up. Raise your elbows in the air and place your palms, face down, on the floor above your shoulders, shoulder-width apart, with your fingers pointing towards your body. Your hands should turn outwards, as in the Peacock balance (see page 51).

With a big inhale and effort, press your hands and feet down into the earth, and lift your tummy up to the sky, arching your back like a bow.

Middle-Stage Variation: Before you attempt to lift your head off the mat, you can rest the crown of your head on the floor between your hands like a tripod, with three points – feet, hands and head – touching the floor.

Now try to straighten your arms and lift your head off the floor, pushing upwards to create a deep arch. Keep your chest area open wide and your feet flat on the floor. Hold the posture for five breaths. Then gently come down to rest and curl up into the Hedgehog, as in step 1.

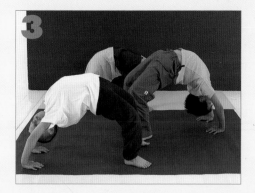

TOPSY-TURVY CRAB

I n this posture, which is an upside-down version of the Crab (see pages 66–7), we are going to join hands and ankles while lying on the tummy, and stretch the body like a bow again. Because crabs are crustaceans – and there are 30,000 species of these many-legged creatures with pincers – they have a hard body case with antennae but no backbone, and we are going to attempt to achieve that feeling of spinelessness with this pose. In addition to easing up the spine, the Topsy-Turvy Crab opens out the chest, or heart, area, as in the Hero pose (see pages 38–9). This area of the body is an extremely important one in yoga, as it relates to both the heart and lungs. As you practise, think about your heart – listening to your heart will help you know yourself better and lead you towards those things that make you feel happy in life. As the Tin Man in *The Wizard of Oz*, who has no heart and cannot feel because he is made of tin, explains:

'You people with hearts have something to guide you,
and need never do wrong; but I have no heart
and so I must be very careful.'

BENEFITS:
The Topsy-Turvy Crab massages the tummy, straightens the back and counteracts slumped shoulders. It tones the waist and helps all bodily functions work well. Like many postures, it is an affirming pose, making you brave and open-hearted!

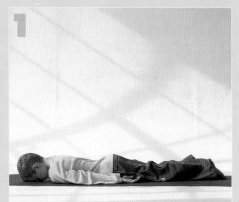

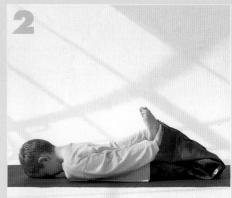

First relax face-down on the floor. Rest with your brow on the mat, unless this squashes your nose – in which case rest one cheek on the mat. Keep your arms lying peacefully by your sides without effort, as if you are resting on the seashore. Your big toes should touch each other and your heels roll outwards.

Carefully bend the knees to raise your feet to the buttocks. Keep your forehead on the floor to relax your neck and to keep the spine straight. Now catch your ankles firmly with both hands, making sure that your knees are hip-width apart. Pull your lower legs into your body, with your heels against your buttocks. Hold for five breaths.

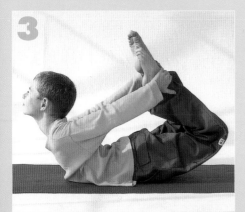

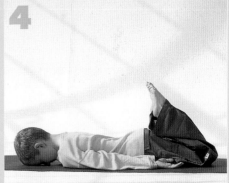

With a big inhale, lift your chest and head, opening out the heart area as you breathe deeply. At the same time, lift your thighs and knees off the ground. Feel the stretch upwards and through your tummy, like a bow being pulled back. Move your knees closer together if you can, as you balance on your bellybutton.

If possible, rock forwards and backwards in the pose, massaging your tummy and swinging, rocking and humming 'MMmmmmmm! MMmmmmmm!' for five full outbreaths. Release your legs, return your arms to your sides, and rest in the sleeping Dormouse pose (see page 80) to relax your back.

ARDHA MATSYENDRASANA
LORD OF THE FISHES

In Sanskrit *matsya* means 'fish', and the story of how this yoga posture came into being goes as follows: Lord Siva, the Hindu god of destiny, went to a lonely island with his wife, Parvati, and beside a river he explained to her the secrets of yoga. Unbeknown to him, a fish popped its head up out of the water to listen. Motionless with concentration, the fish absorbed the teachings. When Lord Siva caught sight of the fish, he sprinkled water over it as a blessing and called it Matsyendra, which means 'Lord of the Fishes'. Fascinated by the practices he'd eavesdropped upon, Matsyendra is said to have swum off and spread the teachings of yoga far and wide.

BENEFITS:
This seated twisting posture is beneficial for the whole torso, helping to relieve backache and tension in the hips. The lower back is released, the abdominal area is massaged and tension in the neck is eased. The liver is stimulated and toned, and so are the intestines and the lower abdomen. Regular practice of the pose also helps firm up and define the waist.

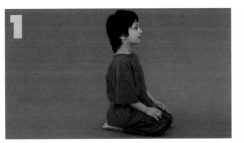

To begin, kneel on the floor with your spine straight, palms flat on your knees and feet tucked under your buttocks. Look directly ahead and take five deep breaths.

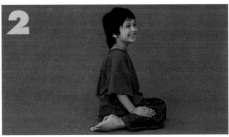

Slide your hips to the left, dropping your left buttock and thigh to the floor, while at the same time sliding both your feet and lower legs out to the right.

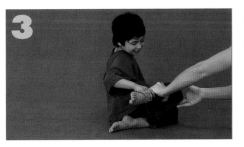

Keeping your chest lifted, clasp your right leg at the ankle. Cross it over your left leg by lifting your right knee and sliding your right foot over your left knee.

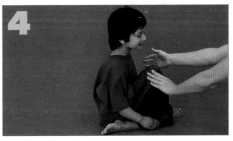

Place your right foot flat on the floor next to the outside of your left thigh, with your bent knee pointing straight up to the sky and your toes pointing forwards.

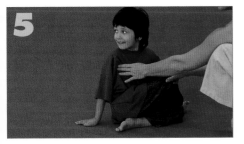

Place your left hand on your right knee and your right hand flat on the floor behind you. Gently twist your torso to the right, lifting your chest to lengthen your torso and deepen the stretch through your tummy and right thigh.

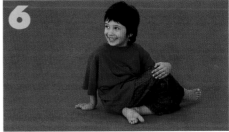

Turn your head to the right and look over the right shoulder. Hug your right knee and breathe freely and deeply, twisting and stretching the spine as much as possible, but without forcing it. Repeat the sequence on your left side.

NAKRASANA
CROCODILE

Like turtles and snakes, crocodiles are reptiles. They have a bony skeleton and scaly skin and most of them lay their eggs on land, although they live both on land and in water in warm climates. They are poached (illegally hunted) for their skins. Like turtles, they need to be protected. You may have heard of a crocodile smile; when a crocodile smiles it is actually panting to let heat escape from its body through its huge mouth. Did you know that after a crocodile has killed and eaten its prey, its eyes water, so that it looks as if it is crying? This is where we get the expression 'crocodile tears'. Another interesting fact is that, in order to lie on the floor of the riverbed, crocodiles will eat stones so that they become heavy enough to sink!

'How doth the little crocodile improve his shining tail,
And pour the waters of the Nile on every golden scale!
How cheerfully he seems to grin, how neatly spread his claws,
And welcome little fishes in with gently smiling jaws!'

LEWIS CARROLL, *ALICE'S ADVENTURES IN WONDERLAND*

BENEFITS:
The Crocodile pose exercises and strengthens the tummy and lower back muscles. Because you are stretching the abdominal muscles, the posture is also good for digestion.

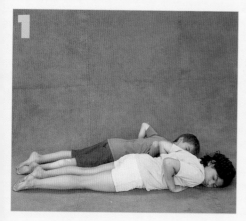

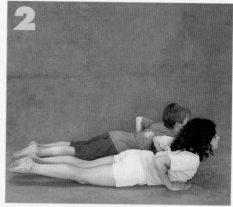

Lie face-down on the floor and press your legs together so that they make one long tail. Point your toes. Press your hands down on the floor beside your chest, with elbows bent. Close your eyes and take five deep breaths. Pretend you are a sleeping crocodile, dozing in the sun, but when you awaken, you will be stretching and on the move!

Now lift your head and upper chest and stretch out your long tail, so that you are balancing on your stomach. Stretch your abdomen as long as you can, as if you are balancing on your bellybutton. Continue to lift up your chest, and take five deep breaths. Point the tip of your tail (your toes) and look forwards into the distance.

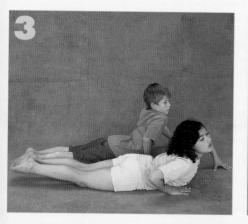

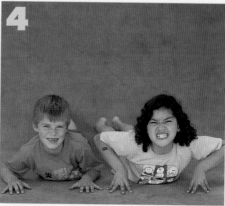

Move along the floor, moving one hand forwards at a time. Can you wriggle forwards on your tummy? Turn your head from side to side, and swing your tail from side to side, too. This is not very easy, so you may need to use your back legs to manoeuvre yourself along. Slink along the floor for five deep breaths.

Now keep very still, take a big breath in, and make the roar of a crocodile as loud as you can, exhaling deeply as you do so. Make a scary crocodile smile by pulling back your lips to show your sparkling white teeth. Show your claws, too, by spreading out your fingers, as if you are marking your territory or protecting yourself from poachers.

KURMASANA TORTOISE

The yogis were fascinated by the tortoise's ability to draw in its limbs and head, symbolizing retreat from temptation. This posture is similar to the Crab (see page 66), because the turtle also carries its shell-house on its back, but here it involves a deep forward bend. It is a fantastic follow-up to the Crab because bending the spine both ways makes it strong and flexible. It is said in yoga that a good healthy back with a lithe, flexible spine leads to long life; and, although they do not bend, tortoises certainly live to be very old. To prepare for the pose, you may like to revisit Aesop's fable 'The Hare and the Tortoise', about a race in which the slow but steady tortoise slowly walks the course without stopping while the proud, quick hare stops to sleep on the way, assuming that it has already won the race. The message here is a good one to consider for your yoga: a slow and steady approach brings success.

BENEFITS:
The Tortoise posture is a great back stretch, tummy massage, hip-opener and brain bath! It refreshes your brain and calms a distracted mind, helping you rest in stillness.

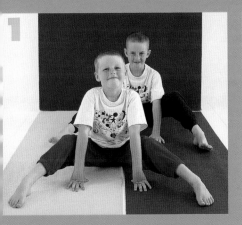

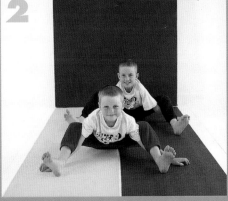

Sit on the floor and stretch your legs wide out in front of you. Bend your knees slightly. Lift your chest and stretch your abdomen, ready for a deep forward bend. Relax your shoulders and smile, because soon you will be folding your limbs around your body to protect yourself from the outside world.

Bending forwards, thread your arms underneath the knees, so your arms stretch sideways under your legs, a bit like a squashed spider. Be careful not to scrunch up your shoulders — aim to coax them under the backs of your knees. Keep your lower abdomen gently curved inwards to protect the stretch in your lower back.

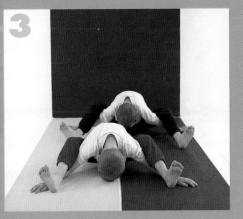

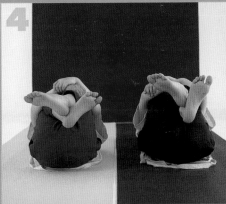

Press your palms down and lower your head, trying to press your shoulders on to the floor. Keep breathing and stretching out your legs and arms for ten deep breaths. Think of this as a deep forward bend, and enjoy the hip-opening stretch. Imagine a protective shell on your back. Close your eyes and 'bathe inwardly' in your little cave.

You are going to return your senses to the outer world now, so slowly gather your legs and arms to your body, clasping your legs with your arms. Roll on to your back into a tiny ball, like a sleeping Hedgehog (see page 23). Curl up, feeling secure, and breathe easily and freely, rocking on your back to massage your torso.

FROG BHEKASANA

Frogs are amphibians, which means they are able to live both on land and in water. Unlike snakes, which are reptiles, they do not have scaly skin; their skin is very thin. They lay their eggs, called frogspawn, in water. Frogspawn look like little black spots surrounded by jelly blobs. As a child I reared frogspawn into tadpoles, mesmerized by the little black spots growing heads and tails, and wriggling out of the jelly to breathe air. Some lose their tails and become frogs, leaving the water to live on land and feed on insects and plants. Here are three Frog poses, which should be followed in sequence. The first is a 'play' posture, then the traditional yoga posture follows, and the final one is for meditation and stillness.

JUMPING FROG

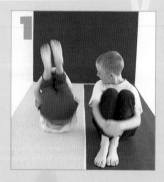
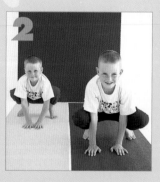
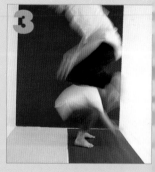

First make sure you are working on a suitably soft mat. From a sleeping Hedgehog (see page 23), start to roll forwards and backwards. Rock until you can roll up on to your feet into a squat position.

Squatting down with knees bent, place your hands on the floor in front of you, and open your eyes wide like a frog. Hold the position, as still as you can, for five deep breaths, in readiness for jumping.

Pretend that the mats are lilypads on a pond and now, with a big breath, leap forwards and try to jump across to someone else's mat, to change places. Leap on an inhale, and exhale when you land.

FROG

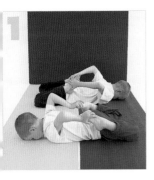 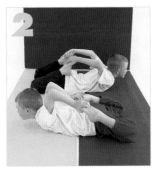 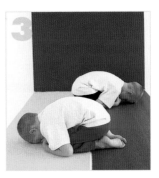

Make sure you have a comfortable mat. Lie face-down with your forehead on the floor and your arms by your sides. Now bend your knees so that your feet rest to the outside of your buttocks, near the hips. Bending the arms at the elbows, lift back and clasp your toes with your fingers. Relax your face and close your eyes, resting for five deep breaths.

Pointing your elbows up to the sky, lift your chest and head up, while at the same time pressing your feet towards your hips with your hands. Keep your knees in line with your hips and do not force them. Hold for five deep breaths. Press gently and breathe deeply, without strain. Aim to press your feet and heels to the outer edges of your hips.

To come out of the posture, let go of your feet carefully and slowly lower your legs to the floor, stretching them out behind you. Draw your face down to the floor, and then fold your body back inwards, gliding smoothly into a kneeling position with your arms tucked around your knees. Curl up into a Dormouse pose (see page 80) for a few quiet breaths.

SITTING OR MEDITATING FROG

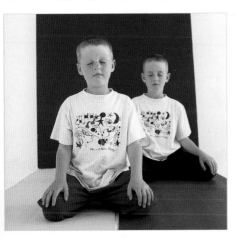

Return to a kneeling position, but keep your knees wide apart. Tuck your feet under your buttocks, with your big toes touching behind you. Place your hands on your knees and make your back very straight, like a reed or a plant stem. Look straight ahead, with eyes closed and at rest, and relax your face. Listen to your breathing, deep into the lower abdomen. Relax your tummy as you breathe, feeling your bellybutton rise and fall.

BIDALASANA CAT

A hundred years ago, there were 100,000 tigers living in the world. Now there are less than 7,000. Each year there are fewer big cats because the jungles and forests are being cut down, so the tigers are losing their habitat. The biggest cats in the world are nearly twice as big as adults, and some are as heavy as four adults! Cats range from these powerful wild animals to tiny defenceless kittens that are carried around by the scruff of their necks in their mother's mouths. Cats can be highly temperamental and solitary, as well as extremely affectionate. Whenever a domestic cat is happy, its tail shoots up in the air and it makes a velvety purring sound. The Cheshire cat in *Alice's Adventures in Wonderland* explains the difference between cats and dogs in the lines below. Look and listen the next time you have a 'conversation' with a cat and a dog to see if it's true.

'You see, a dog growls when it's angry, and wags its tail when
it's pleased. Now I growl when I'm pleased and wag my tail
when I'm angry. Therefore, I'm mad.'
'I call it purring, not growling,' said Alice.

BENEFITS:
This wonderful back stretch arches and flexes the spine, making it free and flexible like a cat's back. The whole torso is stretched, massaged and energized. The back becomes strong and flexible, like a reed beside water, bending in the breeze.

1

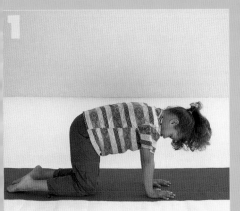

Kneel on all fours, like a cat, with the hands directly beneath your shoulders and the knees beneath your hips. Look down at your hands and press the palms down to the floor, spreading your fingers like starfish. Ground the roots of your fingers (the knuckles) so that you can stretch out your fingers like claws, and with energy.

2

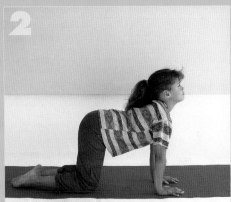

As you inhale, dip your spine down, as if drawing a half-moon with your back. Look up, stretch open the throat area and fill your lungs to the brim. Lift your tailbone as high as you can, pointing it towards the sky. Stretch your tummy, too, and the sides of your waist. Imagine you are smiling from armpit to armpit!

3

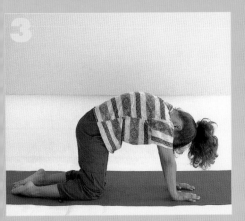

As you exhale, arch your spine up as high as you can, curling your chin in towards your chest, tucking your tailbone under, and stretching your shoulderblades apart. Lengthen the back of your neck by locking your chin tightly onto the little hollow just below your throat, which is called the suprasternal notch.

4

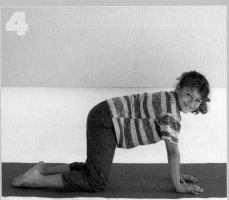

Keep alternating the two movements, using your breath to move you, for ten breaths. Now when you look up, prepare to make the sound of a cat, 'MEEeeeoooooww!'. As you exhale, make the sound last for the whole duration of the outbreath. Do three 'meows'. Now curl up into a Dormouse pose (see page 80) for a short rest.

DOWNWARD DOG

In Sanskrit *adho* means 'downward', *mukha* means 'facing', and *svana* is 'dog'. Dogs are strong, fast hunters and scavengers, and were the first animals to be tamed by humans. The wildest dogs are wolves.

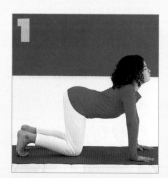

From the arching position of the Cat pose (see step 2, page 79), yawn into a big Downward Dog. Tuck your toes under and then drop your head.

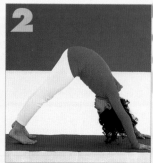

Rise up on to the toes, straightening your legs and pushing your hips to the sky. Take a few big breaths and stretch out your fingers like starfish.

DORMOUSE or CHILD'S POSE

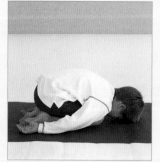

From kneeling, curl up with your eyes closed. Notice how your abdomen rises and falls with each breath.

Now you will become a tiny sleeping dormouse, so sleepy that you are like the dormouse in *Alice's Adventures in Wonderland*, whom the March Hare and Mad Hatter used as an armrest at tea. As you practise the pose, feeling very snug and safe, say to yourself, 'I breathe when I sleep! I sleep when I breathe!'.

RAISED DORMOUSE

You have already discovered the feeling of being topsy-turvy from the Downward Dog (see opposite), where your head drops lower than your heart. Now get the same upside-down sensation by warming up with the Raised Dormouse.

BENEFITS:
The Dormouse and Raised Dormouse poses relax and soothe the body, brain and heart, bringing feelings of security and comfort. The Dormouse is also known as the Child's pose because it echoes the foetal position in the womb, curled up and protected. It is a nurturing posture, and a good one to use whenever you feel overtired or unhappy.

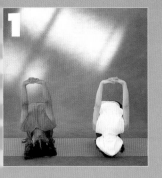 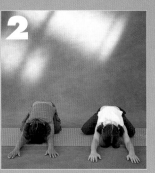 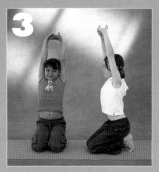

From the Dormouse pose (see opposite), clasp your hands together behind your back. Lift your hips up so that you come on to your knees, and roll from your forehead on to the crown of your head. Lift your clasped arms as high as possible to stretch your shoulders and chest. Take five deep breaths (or three breaths for children under 8 years of age).

On the exhale, return to the sitting Dormouse, but extend your arms out in front of you to stretch out your upper body. Rest there quietly until you are ready to lift up again. Repeat the lift from sitting to rising, with arms extended forward and then clasped behind you, five times, breathing deeply throughout to refresh the lungs, head and heart.

Now lift up to a kneeling position so that your toes are tucked under you. Stretch out the toes and spread the balls of your feet wide. Keep the spine straight and tall. Raise your arms over your head, interlock your fingers and press your palms to the sky for a big stretch. Hold for three breaths, then rest again as in step 2, and repeat.

GOMUKHASANA
COWFACE

In Sanskrit the word *go* means 'cow' and *mukha* means 'face', and this posture is meant to look like the shape of a cow's face! It is a difficult pose, so experiment with your legs and arms separately first if you find it too complicated to do all at once. The pose stretches out the arms and thighs and helps align the upper body.

GOMUKHASANA
LOLASANA
COWFACE LIFT

This lift posture, called the *lolasana*, can be used to change your legs in step 4 of the Cowface pose. In Sanskrit the word *lola* means 'hanging' or 'dangling', and here the body is lifted up to hang between the hands with the legs tucked up, as if you are being lowered into a bath but you don't want to put your toes in the water!

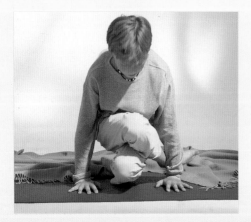

Sit in the Cowface kneeling position (see step 1, opposite). Place your hands on the floor to either side of you, with palms facing down. Press your hands into the floor, and then lift and tuck your body up so that you are hanging between your arms. Hold for one deep inbreath and then lower your body to the floor as you exhale. Now switch legs to repeat the posture on the other side.

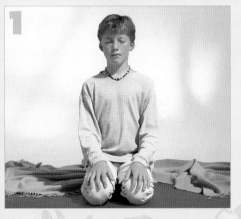

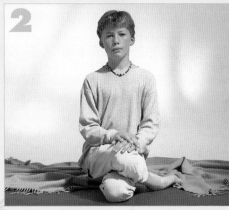

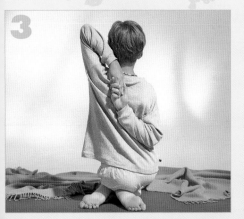

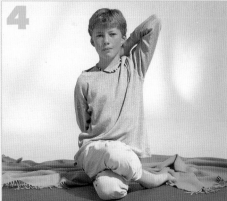

Start in a kneeling position. Sit with the spine alert and straight and your hands resting peacefully on your thighs. With your eyes closed, take five deep breaths in readiness for this calming, meditative posture, which requires focus and balance. The arm and leg joints are manipulated and stretched, so practise carefully.

Wrap your right thigh over your left, almost like crossing your legs. Tuck both feet underneath you, with the toes pointing away, so that you are perched up, with your legs like a chair under you. If your knees hurt or you find it difficult sitting balanced on one leg, or you keep falling over, kneeling is fine. Sit upright with the spine erect.

Lift your left arm up to the sky, bend your elbow and drop your left hand behind your back between your shoulders. Drop your right arm down beside you and then bring your right hand up behind to clasp your left hand. If your shoulders are painful, or the arm position is too difficult, rest your hands on top of each other on your knees.

Hold the position for five to ten breaths, and then gently release your hold, unwind your legs and change sides, so that your left thigh is over your right, your right arm is up, and your left arm is down (see also Cowface Lift, opposite). Hold the stretch, looking straight ahead and keeping steady, and breathe deeply for five to ten breaths.

MALASANA GARLAND

F ragrant garlands, strings of freshly picked sweet jasmine and other exotic flowers, tied together on stems, are often worn in India around the neck, and in this posture the body is woven like a garland. I have a lasting memory of women in bright saris sitting on the pavement in Pune, Maharashtra, in the morning hours among a river of flowers, weaving garlands for the wealthier women to buy and wear for the day – a sea of oranges, pinks and purples mingling in a heady scent.

BENEFITS:
The garland pose strengthens and loosens your back, making it flexible, and massages the tummy. The Lotus mudra is a good hand gesture to practise when you feel lonely or drained.

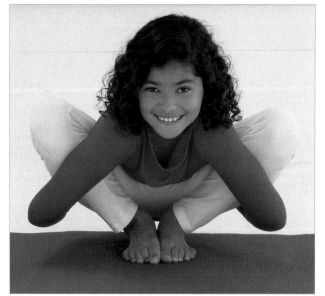

Squat on your haunches, with your feet together and flat, and pressed firmly onto the floor. You are already balancing. Now open the knees wide to the sides so that you reach your chest and upper body forwards through your legs.

On exhale, place your hands on the floor, drawing the shoulders close down towards the floor. Then begin to wrap your arms around your body like a garland of flowers, and see if you can join your hands behind your back and clasp them. This isn't easy, so don't be worried if your fingers don't meet.

If you can, lift your head up and look forward, stretching your back and neck. Balance here for a few deep breaths, as still as you can.

LOTUS
PADMA MUDRA

Flowers grow from the earth, and need deep roots to find nourishment. To finish our earth postures we will make a *mudra*, a hand gesture, that creates the shape of a lotus flower. Think of this as an open-petalled lotus, which floats on muddy waters and sinks its roots deep into the mud, opening its coloured petals up to the sky and sun. You could meditate on the wonder of nature, guided by the words of St Francis of Assisi, who walked barefoot and communed with nature and animals. In his 'Canticle of Brother Sun', St Francis showed his reverence for life by giving thanks for our brother sun, our sister moon and stars, our brothers wind and air, our sister water, our brother fire and our mother earth.

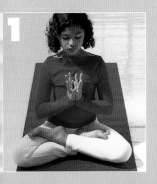

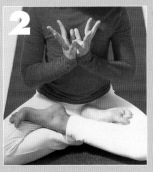

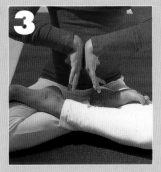

Sit cross-legged, with your feet resting on the thighs if you like (this is known as the Lotus). Hold your hands in front of your heart in prayer position, or *namaste*, the greeting gesture. Keep the base of the hands touching to form a bowl, touching the tips of the little fingers and outer edges of the thumbs.

Now, with a focused mind, open out all your fingers to the sky, like flower petals opening to the sun. Take four deep breaths, imagining you are breathing in the sun. Now breathe in your favourite colour and imagine coloured breath travelling down your throat into your chest.

Now close your fingers into a tight bud, joining the backs of the hands and letting the fingers hang down towards the earth. Feel how your fingers are now like the plant's roots, sinking deep into the earth and drawing nourishment there. Take five deep breaths, then repeat the *mudra*.

WALK THROUGH
THE ANIMALS

Having learned the vocabulary of postures in this section, you now have a language with which you can play. You can make up guided journeys through poses, in which you link one pose to the next, or try the walk-through here, where you metamorphose into different animals. As you alter shape, make the sound of each new animal and change as smoothly as you can, like clay being moulded and brought to life. Feel how different it would be being a wild animal in its natural habitat or a caged animal in the zoo, as described here in the poetry of Judith Nicholls:

'Tiger, eyes dark with half-remembered forest night, stalks an empty cage.'
'Wolf still on his lone rock stares at the uncaged stars and cries into the night.'

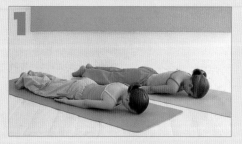

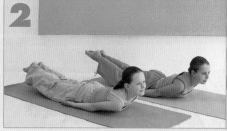

Lie face down on the floor, resting either one cheek on the floor or touching your forehead on the floor. Keep your arms by your sides. Relax and be very still, letting your body sink into the floor like a stone. Imagine you are a sleeping crocodile lying beside a river on a hot, sunny day. Enjoy the feeling of the sun on your back after a long, cool swim. Take five deep breaths.

Waking up, press your legs together to make a tail and lift them off the floor. Bend your arms by your sides and raise your head in the Crocodile pose (see page 73). Make a sound that a crocodile might make with its huge jaws, while remembering the advice of Dr Dolittle: 'Talk to the animals. Walk with the animals! Grunt and squeak and squawk with the animals. And they will talk to you!'

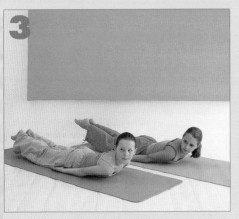

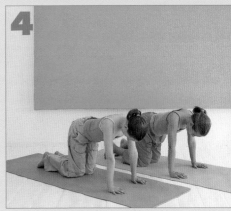

Turn your head from side to side to explore the riverbed, and swing your tail. Try to keep your chest open, your shoulders drawn back and your breathing free and full. Take five deep breaths. If you feel strain in your neck, drop your chin on to your chest for a moment.

Now lower your legs to the floor. Bend your elbows and place your hands, palms down, on the floor, shoulder-width apart. Looking at the floor in front of you, rise up on all fours into the Cat pose (see page 79). Try to keep the movement as fluid as possible.

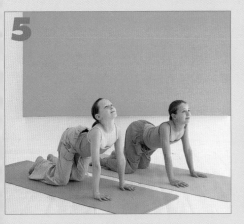

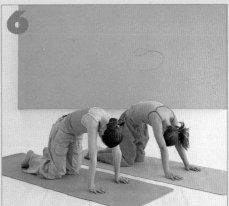

On inhale, look up, open out the chest and stretch your back into a big dip. On exhale, drop your head, look towards your bellybutton and arch your back, pulling your chest in. Alternate the stretches between inhaling, dipping and looking up, and exhaling, arching and looking down, five times. Imagine that you have the flexible spine of a stretching cat.

From a cat you will turn into a dog. On your last cat arch, look up and say 'meeeowww'. Then take a big inhale, and as you slowly breathe out, drop your head between your arms, rise up on your toes and lift your hips skyward into the Downward Dog pose (see page 80). Keep your arms and legs as straight as possible and hold the position, breathing freely.

7

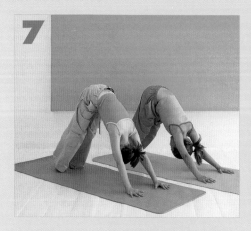

8

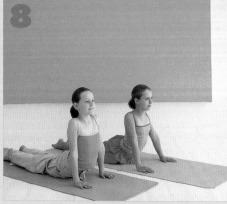

Make the sound of a growling dog, very quietly and steadily. Move in and out of the arching Cat and the Downward Dog, changing shape and sound five times. Return to the Cat arch, then drop your hips between your hands and stretch your legs out behind you.

With hands palms-down, make your arms long and straight to stretch your tummy, lifting and opening your chest into the Cobra (see page 55). Draw your shoulders back and breathe very deeply for five breaths. Now inhale, and as you exhale, say 'sssssssssssssss'.

9

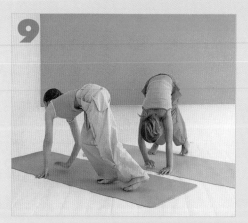

10

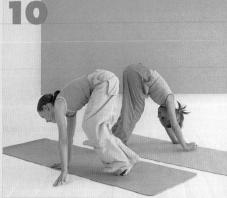

With a deep exhale, push back into the Downward Dog again, raising your hips to the sky. Now bend your knees and walk into the Bear pose (see pages 64–5). Move around the room looking for berries or roots to eat.

Make the sounds of a murmuring bear, 'mmmmmmm', as you pretend to look around in bushes and in holes in the grass, foraging for food. You are a contented, happy bear. Hum a tune. Perhaps you are looking for honey…

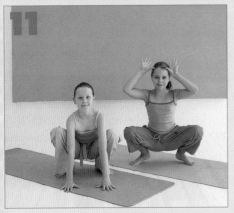

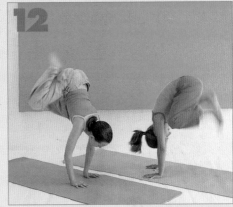

Now you will turn into a rabbit (see Bunny Hops, page 90). Bend your knees and come upright to move out of the Bear pose and into a deep squat. Open your inner thighs to bend the knees out to the sides. Either make your hands into ears or put them on the floor in front of your feet.

Transferring your weight to your hands, bunny-hop up and down, leaping your hips upwards until you land in a squat with your feet resting beside your hands (see page 90). Sniff the air, and put your hands to your ears to listen for sounds of other animals.

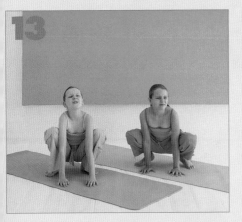

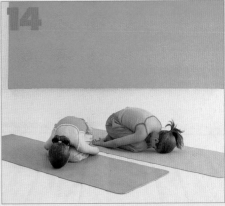

Coming back into a deep squat, place your hands, palms down, on the floor between your feet. Who is in the field? Can you find them? Make sniffing noises as you wrinkle your nose and move your face from side to side.

Now kneel down on your mat, bending forwards to curl up into the Dormouse (see page 80). Keep very still and quiet. Imagine you are a tiny mouse sleeping in the field, 'zzzzzzzzzzz'. Rest for eight deep breaths.

DONKEY KICKS & BUNNY HOPS

Adult supervision is needed to guide the child through these kicks and hops. Before performing the Bunny Hops, you may like to read *The Velveteen Rabbit* by Margery Williams, an enchanting tale of nursery magic, love and what 'real' means.

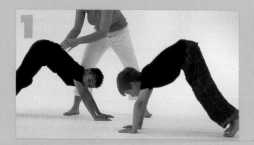

Kneel on all fours as in the Cat pose (see page 79). Then tuck your toes under and lift your hips towards the sky into a Downward Dog (see page 80).

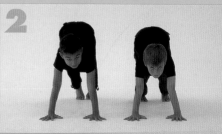

Soften your elbows and knees so that your arms and legs are bent slightly in preparation for kicking like a donkey. Look down, dropping your head between your arms.

Stretch out your back by bending your knees slightly. Now take a little leap off the floor, kicking upwards with one leg at a time, and alternate the kicks. Keep your hips lifted, but make sure that your hands are firmly planted on the floor, like roots, and that both arms are strong, straight and steady so you do not fall over. Repeat ten times on each side.

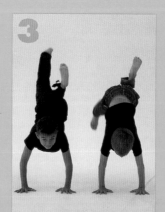

Now do bunny hops. Jump both feet off the floor at the same time in a springing hop, pretending that you are lifting your white tail to the sky, and land back with feet together. Keep your knees bent, and try to inhale as you go into the jumps and then exhale as you land. Repeat ten times. Rest in Dormouse (see page 80) to finish.

URDHO MUKHA VRKSASANA HANDSTAND

Also called the Upward Facing Tree, the Handstand is fantastic for improving circulation and energy levels and giving the brain a boost. Adult supervision is necessary. You'll need lots of energy and the courage of a lion to do this, so get ready.

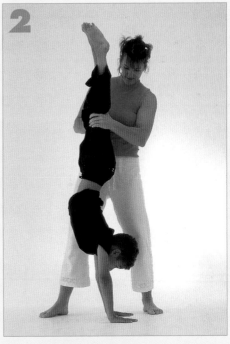

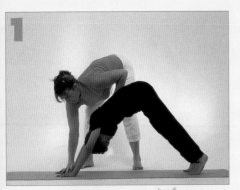

Place your mat next to a wall; the wall will be a safety net for the hops up to the Handstand pose. The adult will need to stand beside you. Face the wall and go into Downward Dog (see page 80), placing your hands firmly on the floor and spreading the fingers out like tree roots. Make your arms straight like pillars. Bend your knees and jump one leg at a time up above your head, so the adult can guide your hips and legs to the wall.

Be careful to keep both arms straight and your body centred so that you do not veer off to one side. Take three deep breaths upside-down, then exhale as you drop your legs down carefully and under control. Hang your torso over your legs with your knees bent and feet firmly planted on the floor, resting in a relaxed Ragdoll forward bend (see page 36). If you are tired, curl up into Dormouse (see page 80) for forty winks before continuing.

SARVANGASANA SHOULDERSTAND

The Shoulderstand, also called the Candle, is a gift to the whole body, mind and spirit. It enables the breathing in of fresh oxygen and the circulation of vital energy, so it's a great posture to do before an exam or competition, or something for which you need courage and focus. The word *sarva* means 'all', or 'whole', in Sanskrit, and *anga* means 'limbs', so this means that the pose benefits all parts of the body. It is essential to have a folded, padded, firm base beneath your shoulders, and an adult will need to supervise throughout to prevent any straining of the neck.

HALASANA MELTING CANDLE

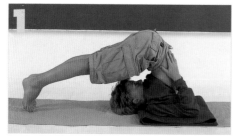 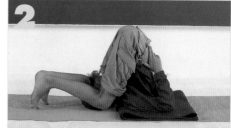

This is also called the Plough. While in the Shoulderstand, imagine your feet as the flame of a candle. Blow out the flame, moving your pointed toes towards your head, and begin to melt your legs down to the floor over your head.

Blow out the candle completely now and bend your knees around your ears. Squeeze your ears with your knees as if you were wearing headphones. Curl up tight and hold for ten breaths before coming out of the pose.

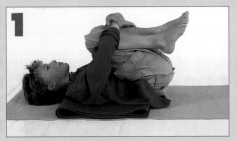

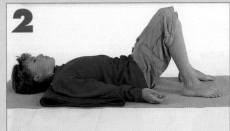

1 Lie down on your back on a padded mat, relaxing the back before you begin. Then clasp your knees to your chest to curl up into a tiny Hedgehog (see page 23).

2 Uncurl, bend your knees and place your feet side by side, tucked up to the buttocks. With your arms alongside your body, press your hands to the floor and open out the chest.

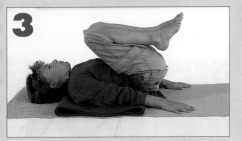

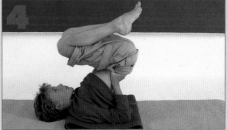

3 Looking straight up with your neck relaxed (no sneaky looks sideways now!), raise your legs up off the mat, tucking them towards your chest. Take two big breaths.

4 Now raise your legs and back up off the floor. Bending your arms at the elbows, support the lower back with your hands. Make sure there is no strain in your back or neck.

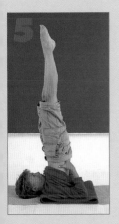

Straighten your legs and press them together like a candle. Straighten your back, supporting it with both hands. With your chin pressed to your chest, listen to your breathing, keeping the breaths very free and steady. Become as still as you can, but breathe in a calm, relaxed way. Rest your eyes and enjoy this topsy-turvy posture for ten deep breaths.

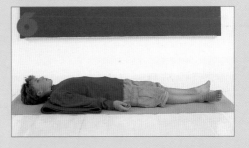

6 When you are ready, bend your legs and uncurl down into the mat again, resting your whole back into the floor. Finally, curl up into a tiny Hedgehog (see page 23) and rock to and fro a little to massage your back.

INCY WINCY SPIDER

I used to enjoy chanting the following rhyme in my bed at night as I walked my legs up the wall into Shoulderstand, and I hope you will, too! In the second line run your legs back down the wall to begin climbing again in the fourth line.

'Incy Wincy Spider climbed up the water spout,
Down came the rain and washed poor Incy out!
Out came the sun which dried up all the rain.
And Incy Wincy Spider climbed the spout again.'

1 Place your yoga mat against the wall. Lie down on your back with your legs resting up against the wall. This is a good way to relax if you are tired, and also a good preparation for a session of yoga, as you can gently stretch out your hamstrings without straining them.

2 As you sing the Incy Wincy Spider rhyme, begin to walk your legs up the wall. When your feet get high enough up the wall, do a Shoulderstand (see pages 92–3), supported by your hands. If you feel unsteady, place your feet back on the wall. Hold for five to ten breaths.

3 Before coming out of the pose, repeat the Melting Candle (see page 92) if you like.

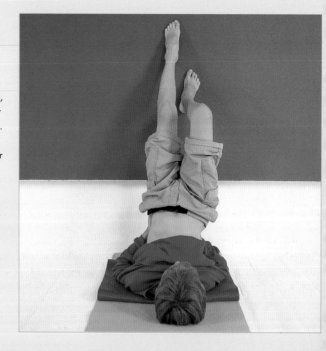

MATSYASANA THE FISH

The Fish is a counterpose to the Shoulderstand (see pages 92–3), and is always practised afterwards because it helps to loosen up and ease the neck and shoulders. Try to flow smoothly from one pose into the other. The word *matsy* means 'fish' in Sanskrit, and it is said that this pose will help you to float on water easily, perhaps because it lifts the chest for deep breathing.

BENEFITS:
The opening up of the throat area encourages deep breathing and expands the chest and lungs. The pose also helps eliminate body waste, relieving constipation. After performing the Fish, rest curled up to release the lower back.

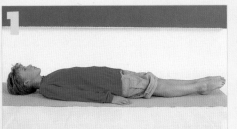

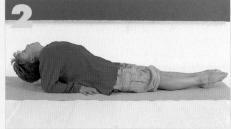

Lie on your back on the floor with your arms alongside your body and palms down. Straighten your legs and press them together, pointing your toes. Relax your face, eyes and brow. Now imagine a jug of warm liquid gold being slowly poured across your forehead, smoothing away any tightness there.

After relaxing for about ten deep breaths, move into *matsyasana*. Lift your upper body to rest on your elbows, pressing your hands by your sides and letting your head drop back. Lift your chest high, so that your back forms an arch like a bridge. Hold the pose for ten deep breaths and then relax to the floor again.

'IT IS ONLY WITH THE HEART THAT ONE
CAN SEE CLEARLY. WHAT IS ESSENTIAL
IS INVISIBLE TO THE EYE.'

ANTOINE DE SAINT-EXUPERY,

THE LITTLE PRINCE

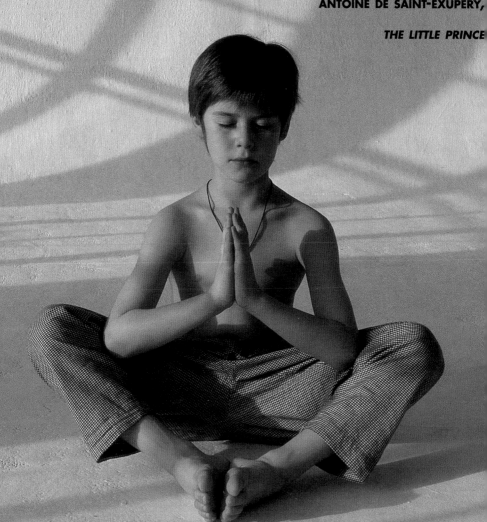

RELAXATION EXERCISES

Before embarking on the relaxation exercises, it is a good idea to tense and stretch out first, so you really get to know the difference between holding in and releasing. Begin with the simple stretches before moving on to guided visualizations. When you tense the body all over, and hold the breath, and then completely let go and relax, you become free from excess physical and mental stresses. Everything becomes simpler, easier and more enjoyable.

STRETCHING STARFISH

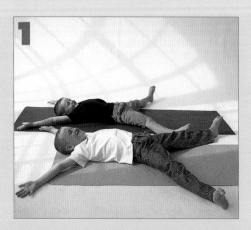

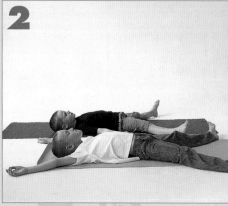

Lie on your back in Corpse pose (see page 22), with your hands at your sides and your feet relaxing outwards. Breathe deeply for five deep breaths. Then inhale and expand your body into a huge, wide starfish, stretching your arms and legs as far as you can reach.

Now, as you exhale, totally relax, becoming completely floppy and loose. Imagine you are like wet seaweed, holding on to nothing at all, just floating on the sea. Breathe deeply for five deep breaths and then return to the Corpse pose. Repeat three times.

SLEEPING STARFISH GAME

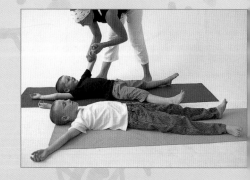

Lie still in a relaxed starfish (see step 2 of Stretching Starfish, above) with your eyes closed, each of you on your own mat. An adult then walks around and lifts an arm here, a leg there, or touches an ear here or a nose there, testing each child for full 'floppiness'. Keep absolutely still, focusing completely on relaxing, or you will be 'out' of the game.

A good way to keep still yet floppy is to concentrate on the ebb and flow of your breathing. Imagine you are floating and the waves are carrying you. Listen to the sound of breath and how it is like the waves of the sea.

SITTING STARFISH

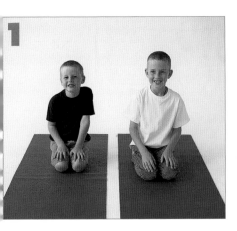

Kneel on your mat with your hands resting on your knees, palms down, and your back straight, looking ahead.

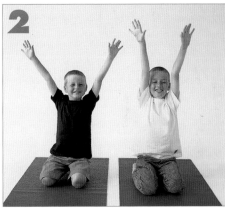

Stretch your arms up over your head, as tall as you can, with the palms opened wide and fingers outstretched.

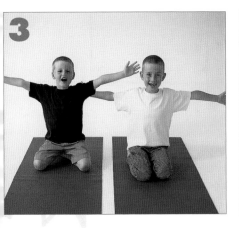

Inhale and stretch your arms outwards in a big starfish. As you exhale, drop your arms back on to your knees and relax. Repeat three times.

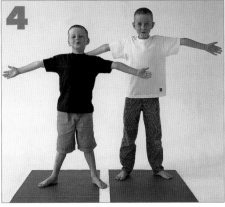

Repeat steps 2 and 3 from a standing position. Start with your feet hip-width apart and pointing outwards and your hands at your sides, and then stretch out on an exhale.

VISUALIZATIONS

Guided journeys and visualizations, practised while you are in a state of deep relaxation, are suitable for all age groups. After leading the child into a 'safe' relaxation, dimming the lights and covering the body with a blanket if necessary, the supervising adult talks through the visualizations as described in the exercises below.

EXERCISE 1: BREATHING WITH IMAGES AND SENSES

1 Lie in the Corpse pose (see page 22). Then close your eyes and begin to create a beautiful picture of a lake, trees and flowers in your imagination. Can you see it? It is a wonderful place to go to for a picnic and you can feel the sun on your back.

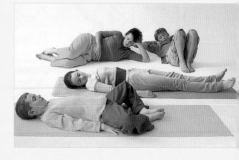

2 Use your breath like a magic wand; as you breathe, the picture becomes clearer and more real. Now look at the colour of the lake. Look at the types of trees around the lake. See the boats on the water. See the flowers at the edge of the lake. What colours are they? See each one: one red, one pink, one yellow, one orange, one blue.

3 One more deep breath and you see the whole picture. Where are you? See the water lapping against the water's edge. Now smell the fragrance of the flowers, the warm air, the breeze… Now feel the water with your fingers – is it warm? Cold? Now hear the sounds around you – what can you hear?

4 Enjoy this beautiful place, surrounded by trees and flowers, the scent of each and every flower. Now say goodbye, as it is time to go home. One… two… three… Goodbye.

5 Very slowly begin to wiggle your fingers and toes. Begin to stretch out your face, and then give a BIG body 'yawn'. Now wake up, fully refreshed, having visited the secret place!

EXERCISE 2: RAINBOW BATHING

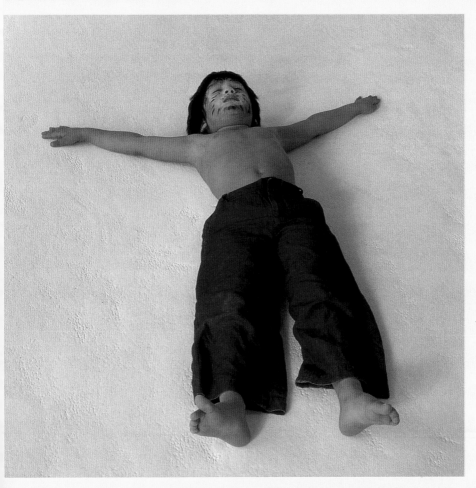

1 Lie in the Corpse pose (see page 22). Then close your eyes and imagine your body is floating like seaweed on water. Breathe deeply.

2 As you lie floating in warm, blue water, imagine there is a broad rainbow above your head. See the rainbow colours as you imagine them to be, one by one, and bathe in each colour: red... orange... yellow... green... turquoise... dark blue... pink... purple... gold.

3 Feel the quality of each colour and breathe it in. Now pick a favourite colour for today and bathe in it for a few moments. (1 minute of silent rainbow bathing.)

4 Very slowly begin to wiggle your fingers and toes. Begin to stretch out your face, and then give a big body 'yawn', stretching out in all directions. Now slowly wake up, fully refreshed, having visited your own special, secret place!

YOGA SLEEP

S imple *yoga nidra* is suitable for all ages and gives children a deep relaxation 'bath', opening up the subconscious and the world of the imagination. Yoga sleep will guide you into a replenishing relaxation where the mind drops from the conscious waking state, with all its ripples of thought waves, anxieties and habits, into the subconscious realm. Here the body, mind and emotions are recharged, knowledge is increased, memory is enhanced, and you will emerge refreshed and renewed. An invaluable way for adults to relieve stress, the technique is a wonderful one to introduce to children, but keep the practice short, to ten minutes, as children tend to go 'deeper' than adults. The three-step process below will take you from breathing, through a body scan – which helps children identify body parts as well as visualize them and develops stillness and attention – to the relaxation.

FOLLOW-ONS FROM RELAXATION

This is a good time to move on to quiet activities, taking advantage of the relaxed and contemplative state of the children. You may like to do some of the following:

- Read a story or make up your own. You could take turns telling a story, or each person could contribute a sentence to make up a story.
- Talk about the yoga session during circle time (see page 123).
- Make up a positive phrase, called a *sarkalpa*, to repeat to yourself, and which calms you and makes you happy.

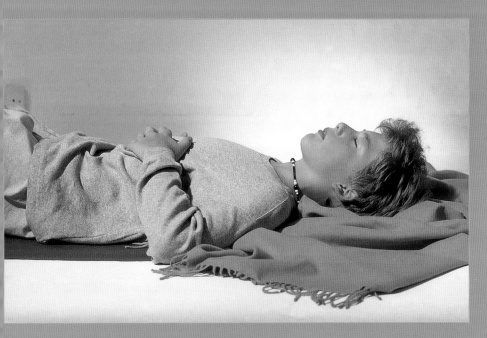

RELAXED BELLY BREATHING

1 Sit cross-legged with the back straight or lie down flat on your back. Breathing deeply, imagine a paper boat is on your tummy, rising and falling with the wavelike breaths (see page 108). Feel your bellybutton rise with your inbreath and fall with your outbreath. Take five deep breaths.

2 Every time you exhale, say to yourself in your head or whisper 'peace'. Repeat five times. Now choose a word of your own that makes you feel happy and calm – just one word, rather than a phrase. Concentrate on your word for five outbreaths. Alternatively, you can say the word aloud.

BODY SCAN

1 Now, like a butterfly alighting on different parts of the body, draw your attention to each part of the body as the grown-up names it, from the toes, ankle, foot, knee, hip and upwards, until the adult has talked through the whole of the right side of the body. Take a few moments to concentrate on relaxing each body part.

2 Repeat on the left side of the body, starting from the toes and finishing with the head and the 'sense organs' (the ears, eyes, nose, mouth and tongue).

IN THE ZONE

1 In the resulting state of deep rest, visualizations, such as Rainbow Bathing, can be tried (see pages 100–1). Allow a maximum of 10 minutes for this.

2 To awaken gently, bring awareness back to the room, as well as to the body. The adult can begin to open blinds or curtains if they have been closed. Little by little begin to stretch, starting with toes and fingers and gradually working into a whole body 'yawn'. Then roll over on to one side for a few moments before sitting up.

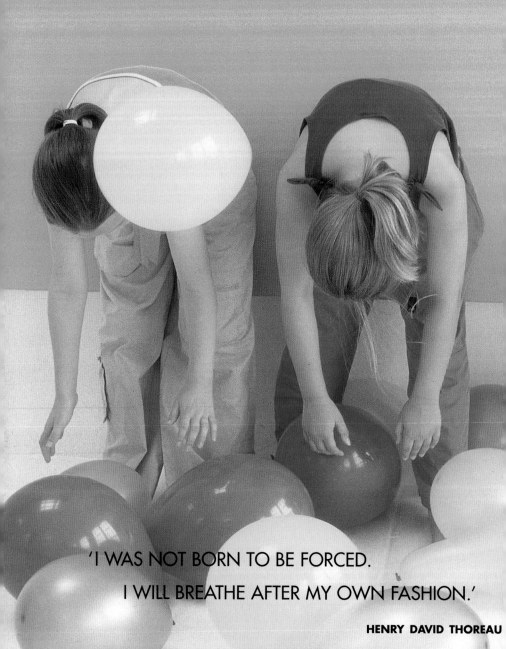

'I WAS NOT BORN TO BE FORCED.

I WILL BREATHE AFTER MY OWN FASHION.'

HENRY DAVID THOREAU

SENSE EXERCISES & BREATHING

In his book *The Secret of Happy Children*, Steve Biddulph recommends that children receive a diet of regular sense stimulation in order to thrive and grow. The ingredients of this 'diet' can be included in a yoga session through games and exercises that awaken the senses of touch, taste, sight, sound and smell. Yoga exercises are challenging and contemplative, and always link, rather than separate, the mind and body.

LISTENING

The term *antar mouna* means 'inner silence', and in this practice the mind is focused on sensations and thoughts in order to become alert and sensitive. In this exercise, encourage the child to feel safe, calm and still, but not to fall asleep!

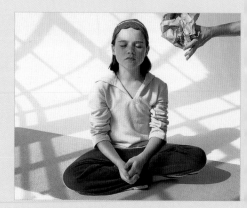

1 The adult makes three different sounds, perhaps clicking the tongue, crunching a paper bag, splashing the hands in water, cutting open an apple, or using recordings from nature, such as birds or wild animals, pausing between each sound. Repeat the three sounds three times (remember children like repetition). Ask the children to identify or describe each sound.

2 Now repeat the sounds at different distances from the children. Invite them to listen to the sounds that are farthest away. Then ask them which sound is closest. Ask if they hear a sound between these two. Then ask the children to identify each sound.

TRATAK SEEING

Tratak, gazing at one point, helps to build concentration and memory. The adult can keep time during the session, and must be present when a candle is used.

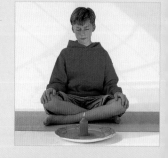

1 Use a candle flame as the gaze-point, sitting 90 cm (3 ft) away and watching the flame. After 1 minute, close your eyes for another minute and try to see the flame again with the mind's eye. Open your eyes and repeat.

2 Using a computer, print out the word 'joy' in bold letters, half-filling an A4 page, with a black dot in the centre of the 'o'. Sitting with your back straight, hold the paper out at arm's length in front of you and gaze at the dot fixedly for 1 minute. Now close your eyes for a second, open them again, and see the dot. Where is it? Repeat the exercise, but keep your eyes closed for 1 minute. What do you see?

VIEWING

Repeat each of the following steps five times, followed by the Near and Far Viewing. Performed slowly, these exercises revitalize and tone the eye muscles.

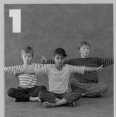

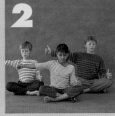

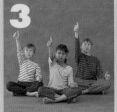

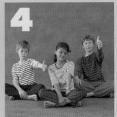

Sideways: With arms wide and thumbs up, look at the right thumb, up at the centre of your brow, then the left thumb. Return left to right.

Diagonal: Move your left fist to your left knee. Focus on the right thumb, then switch to the left. Close the eyes for 1 minute. Change sides.

Up and Down: Place both fists on your knees. Lift the right thumb high, following with your eyes, then back down. Change sides.

Rotational: Draw a wide circle in the air with one thumb, following with the eyes, first clockwise, then back. Change sides.

NEAR AND FAR VIEWING

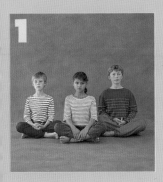

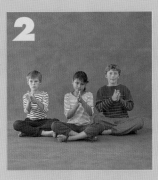

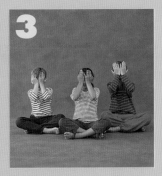

Resting your hands in your lap, focus your eyes on the nose tip (very near), and then focus on a distant object. Switch back and forth three times.

To finish the viewing exercises, palm your eyes. To do this, warm up your hands by rubbing them vigorously together for a few moments.

Close your eyes, relax, and place your warmed hands over your eyes. Hold for a few moments and then repeat three times.

BREATHING PRACTICES
FOR ALL AGES

B reathing gives oxygen to the blood, which fuels the body's cells and removes carbon dioxide. Trees and plants do the opposite, absorbing carbon dioxide and producing oxygen, which is why our forests are essential to sustain all life. Breathing deeply and freely will help to keep you relaxed and healthy. The following exercises will help you to explore the action of breathing through sight and sound.

PAPER BOATS

Using a paper boat as a tool, we can see the movement of the breath, like waves, in the tummy, which allows the child to become aware of their abdomen and their breathing. This exercise releases tension around the navel.

Lie on your back on the floor with your eyes closed and arms completely relaxed. Place a paper boat on your tummy and feel it rise as you inhale, and then fall as you exhale, like a boat on the waves of the sea.

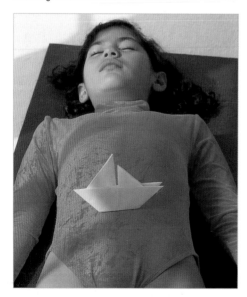
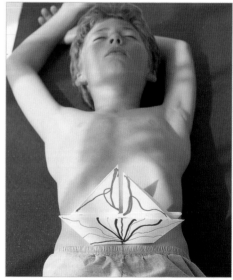

BLOWING UP A BALLOON

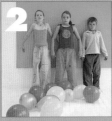 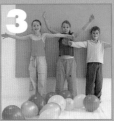 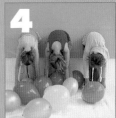 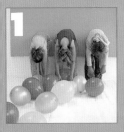

Stand in a relaxed forward bend (see Ragdoll, page 36), and relax your back. Imagine you are a weeping willow tree. When the adult comes to touch you, move like a tree in the wind.

Now begin to blow up like a balloon with each breath. As you inhale, rise a little and stop. As you inhale again, rise a little more and stop. Repeat until you are as tall as an oak tree.

Now stretch your arms out like the branches of a tree. If you like, you can do a modified Tree pose (see page 29), with one leg crossed over the other at the ankle.

Now you burst – pop! – like a balloon. Collapse down to a floppy weeping willow tree again, and imagine that you are trailing your branches (arms) and twigs (fingers) in the water.

VARIATION

Repeat steps 1 to 3 above, but this time deflate breath by breath. As you blow out, begin to deflate, and stop. Take a big breath in, and then slowly blow out, dropping a little more, and stop. Continue until you are fully collapsed like a burst balloon. Repeat the whole sequence three times.

HA! HA! HA! BREATHING

Adding sounds to outbreaths helps self-confidence and self-expression, develops pronunciation and strengthens abdominal muscles, which engage when we communicate. To release tension try Ha! Ha! Ha! breathing. As you inhale and exhale in a pose, add a 'ha!' sound as you exhale to express excess energy.

BEE BREATH

The bee breath, humming 'mmmmmm', is the only specific breathing exercise to give to little ones under 8 years, as their lungs are still forming. This breathing practice will calm anger, soothe anxiety and improve the vocal cords.

Sit cross-legged with the spine straight as a flute or a reed by a riverbank. Part the teeth, but keep the mouth closed. Close both ears with your index fingers. Exhale with a gentle 'hummmmm' sound, slowly and steadily. Repeat five times.

BREATHING PRACTICES
FOR OVER-8S

At eight years old, the alveoli, minute air sacs that look like bubblewrap in the lungs, stop growing in size, but not in number. This is the ideal time to introduce structured breathing techniques in order to train the cardiovascular and respiratory (heart and lung) systems. The following breathing exercises should never be forced or uncomfortable, and only be introduced with ease and relaxation in an environment that has fresh air circulating.

STRUCTURED PRANAYAMA: ALTERNATE-NOSTRIL BREATHING

This exercise, which channels the breath in and out through alternate nostrils, is said to balance the left and right sides of the brain, and to induce a natural calm. It also maintains good condition of the pineal gland (see page 17). Always follow the adult's guidance, and do not strain your breaths. Practise to become comfortable with this breathing technique, never forcing the breath but breathing smoothly and easily. It is a good idea to count during the inhalations and exhalations – learning rhythmic breathing and pacing yourself will nurture discipline.

BENEFITS:
In pranayama basic breathing techniques, the lungs are strengthened and cleansed, and the nadis (energy channels) are purified, which increases prana (vital air) intake. As the length of each exhalation is increased, stale air is eliminated. The deepening of inhalations increases oxygen uptake. Slowing down the breath stills the mind.

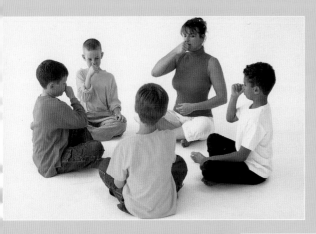

1 Sit cross-legged on the floor with your back as straight as possible, your sitting bones grounded and your chest area open with your shoulders back. Breathe freely.

2 Rest your left hand on your lap, or curl in the index and middle fingers to touch the thumb tip, making the traditional *mudra* gesture to calm the senses. The right thumb will be used to close the right nostril along the right side of the nose, and the fourth finger of your right hand will be used to close the left nostril along the left side of the nose. The left hand will remain in your lap (unless you are left-handed, in which case you will be resting your right hand in your lap).

3 Inhale through both nostrils. Close the right nostril with the thumb, and exhale through the left nostril. Count to four. Inhale through the left nostril. Count to four.

4 Close the left nostril and exhale through the right nostril to the count of four. Inhale through the right nostril to the count of four.

5 Close the right nostril and exhale through the left nostril to the count of four. Inhale through the left nostril to the count of four.

6 Release the left nostril and exhale completely. This is one round. Repeat this alternate-nostril breathing sequence to practise ten whole rounds.

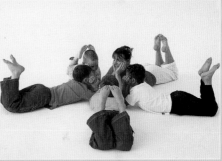

VARIATION WITH LEGS

1 To introduce *pranayama* like a game, lie face-down in Crocodile pose (see page 73), resting on your elbows with your palms cupping the cheeks.

2 As you inhale, raise your right leg at the knee and imagine breathing in through the right nostril. As you breathe out, lower your right leg and imagine breathing out through the right nostril.

3 On your second inhale, raise your left leg at the knee and imagine breathing in through the left nostril. As you breathe out, lower your left leg and imagine breathing out through the left nostril.

4 Repeat step 2, but raise both legs at the same time.

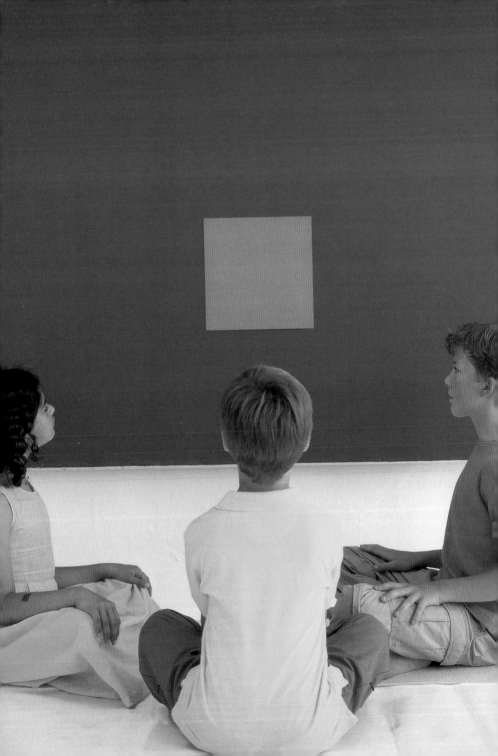

YANTRA BREATHING

A yantra is a pattern, often geometrical, that helps the mind to concentrate and focus during breathing and meditative sessions. By having a tangible symbol, in this case a square or a circle, we can help to connect with the invisible essence of the breath. This calming and centring exercise concentrates the mind.

BREATHING WITH A SQUARE

You can do this exercise by visualizing a square in your mind's eye, but first practise it by using a drawing of a square. We use the square to practise moving the breath along its edges. This is a good example of how the mind and body are linked through breathing with awareness.

1 Draw a 30-cm (12-in) square on paper, or cut out a square from coloured paper. Tape the square to a wall at eye level, or hold it out in front of you. Sit in a comfortable cross-legged pose with your spine straight and gaze at the square.

2 Look at the bottom-left corner of the square, inhale, and trace the line with your eyes to the top-left corner.

3 Exhale, following the line with your eyes and breath from the top-left corner to the top-right corner.

4 Inhale, following the line with your eyes and breath from the top-right corner to the bottom-right corner.

5 Exhale, following the line from the bottom-right corner to the bottom-left corner. Repeat five times.

BREATHING WITH A CIRCLE

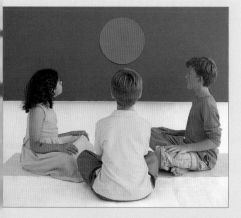

1 In the same way as in the square exercise, above, draw a circle on paper, or cut out one out from coloured paper, measuring about 30 cm (12 in) in diameter. Tape it to a wall at eye level, so you can see it from a comfortable sitting position.

2 Gaze at the circle. Starting at the 9 o'clock point of the circle, inhale, following the edge clockwise from left to right, tracing a half-moon arc to 3 o'clock.

3 Exhale, following the line in a bottom half-moon arc from 3 o'clock back to the 9 o'clock starting point. One complete breath (in and out) completes a cycle. Repeat five times.

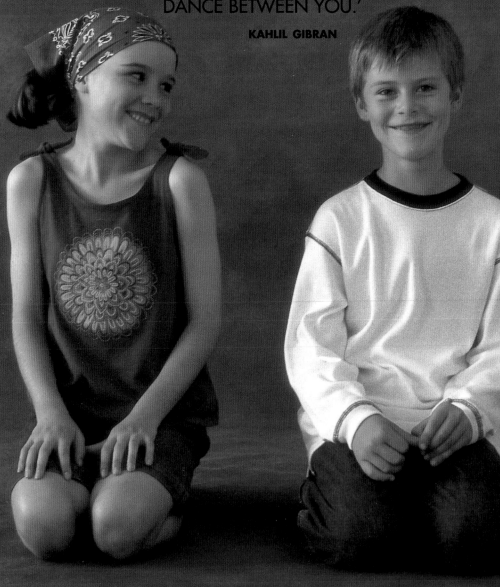

'BUT LET THERE BE SPACES
IN YOUR TOGETHERNESS,
AND LET THE WINDS OF THE HEAVENS
DANCE BETWEEN YOU.'

KAHLIL GIBRAN

GROUP & PARTNER EXERCISES

Practising yoga with others develops self-control, social awareness and spatial dynamics. It teaches children how to interact and connect with others and how to appreciate differences. The games and postures shown here can be adapted, reinvented and added to. They are also sense exercises, which aim to encourage coordination, sensitivity, perception, attention and creative thinking. As an extra benefit, integrate the suggestions for guided play on pages 12–13.

TREES IN THE WIND

Here we explore how balance, rooting our feet and legs into the earth, can help us remain steady, sure and stable, regardless of what is happening around us.

1 The supervising adult divides the group of children into two: one half will be a forest of trees and the other half will be the wind. The trees stand in Tree pose (see page 29), still and steady, making sure there is space around each one for roots to grow freely.

BENEFITS:
Balance, coordination and mental focus (mind control) are cultivated in games like this one. The exercise will help you to find inner stability in the midst of chaos.

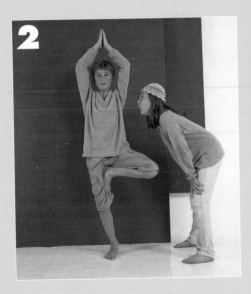

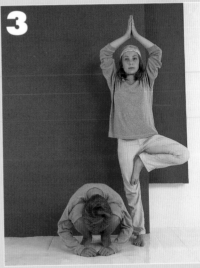

The wind group runs around blowing, singing 'oooooooohhhhhhh', and stopping at different trees. The adult then asks the wind children to try to blow the trees over, but without touching them. The trees must remain as still and focused as they can in their poses, with their faces like statues.

Next the adult says 'all change', so that the trees drop into seeds (tiny and curled-up, like a squatting version of the Dormouse, see pages 80–1), and freeze. The wind children now become steady new trees. The seeds then grow tall to turn into wind and blow around the trees, repeating the exercise.

MIXING BOWL

This exercise is good for developing and improving coordination and trust between the partners, and can be as useful for adults as for children. The aim here is to imagine yourselves as one unit, working in harmony to 'mix the bowl'.

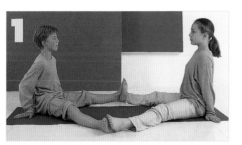

The adult divides the group into pairs. Face your partner and stretch your legs out straight, as wide as you can. Form a square with your four legs, with the soles of your flexed feet pressing against each other. Rest the palms of your hands on the floor.

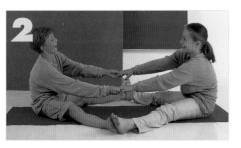

Clasp hands with your partner and, keeping your arms straight, begin to stir a circle round and round, as if you are mixing a huge pot of dreams. Ensuring that both you and your partner circle in the same direction will take coordination.

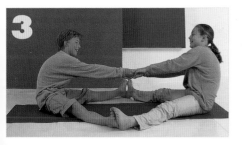

Keep circling from side to side and forwards and backwards, trying to keep the movement fluid. Think about what is in your pot: hot porridge or fruit punch? You decide, and tell the adult when she comes to check your cooking.

WRITING ON THE B(L)ACKBOARD

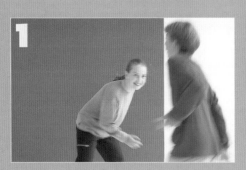

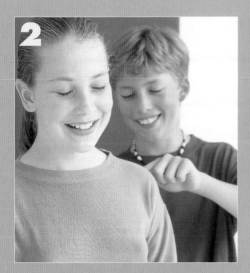

The adult divides the group of children into two: As and Bs. Choose two animal or warrior poses, such as the Cobra and Warrior. Remember the first letter of each: C and W. On the command 'go', run around the room and on the command 'freeze', stop.

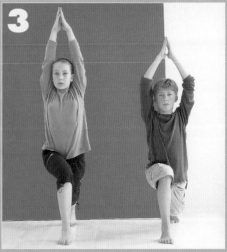

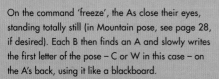

On the command 'freeze', the As close their eyes, standing totally still (in Mountain pose, see page 28, if desired). Each B then finds an A and slowly writes the first letter of the pose – C or W in this case – on the A's back, using it like a blackboard.

The As then assume the pose indicated on their backs, and the Bs freeze in the same pose. Hold for five deep breaths. Now advance to Cleaning the B(l)ackboard, see opposite, step 1, to rub out the letters. Choose new poses after a few rounds.

CLEANING THE B(L)ACKBOARD

This second part to the b(l)ackboard game focuses on learning about trust, safety and similarity through direct contact, coordination and mirroring techniques.

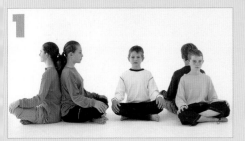

1 Sit cross-legged on the floor with your partner, back to back, and nestle close together. Wriggle in so that you rub out the letter on your b(l)ackboard.

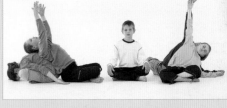

2 Now one partner leans forwards, while the other leans back. Take five breaths and reverse positions. Repeat three times. You can also do this as a sideways mirroring stretch.

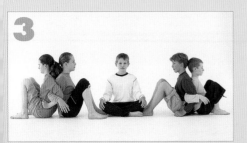

3 Remaining back to back, bend your knees with your feet flat on the floor. Interlock your arms at the elbows for stability. You are now going to try to rise to your feet together, but first rock sideways back and forth a little to get used to working as one in this position.

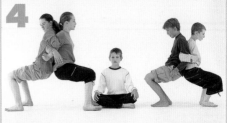

4 Pressing firmly back-to-back (and trusting each other!), aim to lift up to a standing position together. You will find it helpful to keep your lower backs in contact and to inch your feet in gradually as you rise. Once you are standing, release your arms and stretch them to the sky.

MAKING BRIDGES

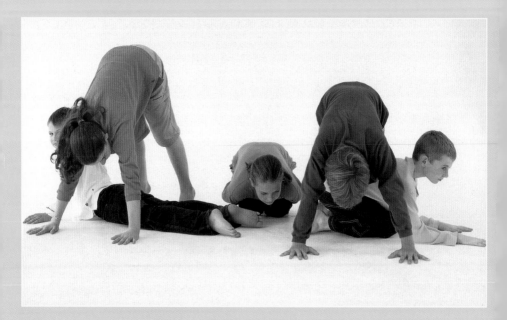

All varieties of animal can be called on to play this metamorphosis (changing) game, but keep the Downward Dog to provide a bowing arch or 'bridge', under which the other animals can crawl. The Crab, or upward-facing bow, (see pages 66–7) can also be used as a 'bridge' but may be a trickier pose for children to hold for long. Refer to the Creatures of the Sky, Water, Wild and Earth in Chapter 3 to choose your animals and see how you might metamorphose from one another.

1 The adult organizes the group into dogs (Downward Dog, page 80), mice (Dormouse, pages 80–1) and snakes (Cobra, pages 54–5). On calling out the names, each child assumes their given pose.

2 On the command 'go' the mice and snakes crawl under the dogs. Mice make the sound 'eeeee! eeeee!' and snakes make the sound 'sssss! sssss!'. The children can then swap poses for another game of Making Bridges.

GRANDMA'S FOOTSTEPS

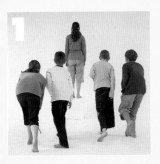

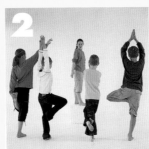

Yoga postures are used in this classic game, where children creep up on 'grandma'. When the person at the front of the room turns round, the other children, who are inching their way forwards, freeze into yoga postures. Anyone who moves is 'out'. Alternatively, the 'grandma' can call out a posture, which all the other children must quickly adopt.

FROZEN STATUES

Yoga games develop self-awareness in children, and also train, discipline and coordinate both mind and body. Many classic children's games, like the ones shown here, can include yoga postures to extend the challenge.

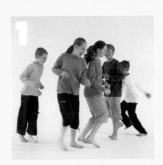

This is another children's game that incorporates yoga postures. Play music, letting the children dance around the room. Then stop the music and call a posture: the children must immediately freeze into that pose.

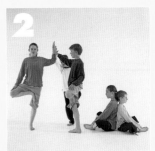

Children can then group together to create a posture sculpture. Some examples may be: two Warriors touching, Trees linking arms, standing forward bends with backs touching, and Butterflies sitting back to back.

CLOSING PRACTICES

Specific activities, such as poetry readings, visualizations or 'sharing' sessions, can be used to mark the end of the yoga class. In this 'closing time' you could also try kirtan, the practice of engaging in song. Just sing a simple song and get the children to sing it back. A song containing different languages can be particularly valuable, helping you to tap into the subconscious and stimulate less-conditioned responses. You may also like to play percussion instruments or other noisemakers.

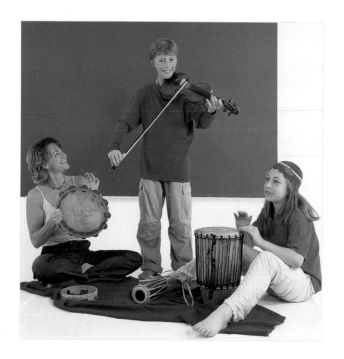

'Listen to the children,
they are wise.
Give them a language
to express themselves.'

CHRIS WADE, *HEADTEACHER,*
WINNS PRIMARY SCHOOL

CIRCLE TIME

Sitting together in a circle is a perfect way to end a session of yoga, or indeed any activity. It will encourage sharing, bring a feeling of unity, and cultivate imagination and calmness. The group pose here creates a geometrical pattern and the exercise is a circle form of Alternate-Nostril Breathing (see pages 110–11).

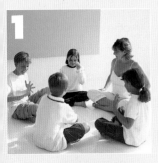

Seated in a circle, hold hands with left hands turned upwards and right hands turned downwards to make a chain, linking hands.

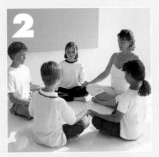

Close your eyes and breathe very peacefully, imagining that you are inhaling through your left hand and exhaling through your right hand.

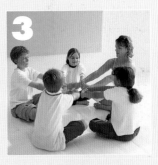

Now open your eyes and reach towards the middle of the circle. Clasp hands with the others in your group, keeping your shoulders relaxed.

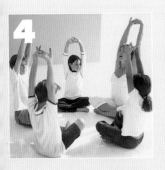

Inhale and reach to the sky, fingers interlocked and palms facing up.

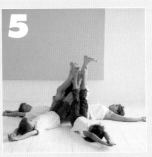

Now relax on your back and make a sculpture by interweaving your legs.

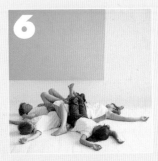

Imagine that the wind is blowing the sculpture over, and flop. Sleep...

RESOURCES

GLOSSARY

Ahimsa nonviolence

Antar mouna inner silence

Asana steady posture, balance, poise

Ashram house of spiritual retreat

Dharana concentration

Eka-grata one-pointed focus, using body, mind and imagery

Guided journeys imaginative talk-through to help soothe and create a calm state

Guna an attribute, quality; the universe is composed of three gunas – rajas, sattva and tamas

Guru a spiritual teacher; a carrier of light

Karma the law of universal cause and effect; action or deeds which lead one towards or away from bliss; yoga of unconditional service

Kirtan simple positive song with others

Mandala a mystic circular diagram used for concentrating cosmic and psychic energy

Mantra a Sanskrit syllable, a sacred sound or phrase used to concentrate energy

Metta a buddhist term for loving kindness

Mudra a gesture to concentrate energy, usually done with the hands

Nadi energy channel in the subtle body

Nadi shodana alternate-nostril breathing

Namaste the universal prayer position, a hand mudra

Om mystical syllable signifying the source of all things; similar to the Christian 'Amen'

Prana inner energy or vital air

Pranayama the Fourth limb of yoga, the science of breathing

Rajas the quality of stimulation, passion; one of the three gunas

Sattva the quality of balance, truth, vitality; the pure guna

Shambhavi mudra a gesture or gazing that concentrates on the centre of the brow to stimulate intuition and perception

Shiva male god in Hindu mythology

Tamas the quality of inertia or lethargy; one of the three gunas

Vipassana silent retreat or in-sight meditation

Visualization the conscious creation and crystallization of images with the mind's eye; imagining

Yantra a geometrical symbolic aid to contemplation

Yoga nidra yogic sleep or deep relaxation

YOGA CENTRES & ORGANIZATIONS

The Art of Health
280 Balham High Road
London SW17 7AL
tel 020 8682 1800
www.artofhealth.co.uk
runs teacher training and kids'
Yoga Bugs classes

Bihar School of Yoga
Mungar, Bihar
811 201, India

British Wheel of Yoga
1 Hamilton Place
Boston Road, Sleaford
Lincs NG34 7ES
tel 01529 306 851
www.bwy.org.uk

Iyengar Yoga Institute
223a Randolph Avenue
London W9 1NL
tel 020 7624 3080
www.iyi.org.uk

The Life Centre
15 Edge Street
London W8 7PN
tel 0207 221 4602
www.thelifecentre.org

Light on Yoga Association
www.loya.org.uk

Sangam
Gingi Lee & Liz Lark
80b Battersea Rise
London SW11 1EH

Satyananda Yoga Centre
70 Thurleigh Road
London SW12 8UD
tel 020 8673 4869

Vini-Yoga Britain
www.viniyoga.co.uk
for listings of Viniyoga
practitioners

Yoga Biomedical Trust
Royal Homeopathic
Hospital Trust
60 Great Ormond Street
London WC1N 3HR

Yoga Therapy Centre
90–92 Pentonville Road
London N1 9HS
tel 020 7689 3040
www.yogatherapy.org

RETAIL/MULTIMEDIA

Yoga-Mad
20c Pershore Trading Estate
Pershore, Worcs
WR10 2DD
tel 01386 555 955
www.yogamad.com
for yoga mats

Sweaty Betty
1 Beak Street
London W1F 9RR
tel 020 7287 5428
www.sweatybetty.com
for yoga clothing

'Peter and the Wolf', Compact Disc. Sergei Prokofiev (composer), Richard Stamp (conductor), Academy of London (orchestra), Sir John Gielgud (narrator), Virgin 7243 5 61137 2.

'The Young Person's Guide to the Orchestra', Compact Disc. Benjamin Britten (composer and conductor), Polygram 47509.

India: The Kingdom of the Tiger, film documentary on Jim Corbett's fight to save the Bengal tiger, Chris Palmer (producer), Keero Singh Birla (writer), Bruce Neibaur (director), released 2002.

USEFUL WEBSITES

www.childrensyoga.com
www.healthypages.net
www.lizlark.com
www.natural-healing.co.uk
www.nwf.org
    (national wildlife federation)
www.yogaclass.net
www.yogainside.org
www.yogajournal.com
www.yogasite.com
www.yoga-wise.com
www.yogiway.com

BIBLIOGRAPHY &
SUGGESTED READING

Arundhati, compiler, Yoga Education for Children – A Manual for Teaching Yoga to Children. Satyananda Paramahansa International, 1984. (available from the Satyananda Yoga Centre)

Attenborough, Liz, When All the World's Asleep: A Children's Book of Poems and Prayers, Element, 1998.

Barks, Coleman, translator, The Essential Rumi, Penguin, 1999.

Biddulph, Stephen, The Secret of Happy Children, HarperCollins, 1999.

Blake, William, Songs of Innocence and Experience, Oxford University Press, 1967.

Carle, Eric, The Very Busy Spider, Hamish Hamilton, Penguin, 1984.

Carroll, Lewis, Alice's Adventures in Wonderland, Puffin, 1946.

Currey, Anna, illustrator, The Macmillan Treasury of Nursery Rhymes and Poems, Macmillan, 1998. (Celia Warren, 'Roly Poly Bear' excerpt, page 64)

Dewhurst-Maddock, Olivea, The Book of Sound Therapy: Heal Yourself with Music and Voice, Gaia Books, 1993.

Duff, L, editor, Aesop's Fables: A Children's Treasury, Tiger Books, 1993.

Foster, John, editor, Another Second Poetry Book, Oxford University Press, 1988.

French, Vivien, and Paul, Korky, Aesop's Funky Fables, Puffin Books, 1999.

Gibran, Kahlil, The Prophet, Heineman, 1980.

Iyengar, B K S, Light on Yoga, Aquarian Press, 1991.

Johnson, Robert A, He: Understanding Masculine Psychology, HarperCollins, 1989. (traditional Zen saying, excerpt, page 7)

Kabat-Zinn, Jon, Wherever You Go, There You Are: Mindful Meditation in Everyday Life, Hyperion, 1994.

Khalsa, Shakta Kaur, Fly Like a Butterfly: Yoga for Children, Rudra Press, 1998.

Landaw, Jonathan and Brooke, Janet, Prince Siddhartha: The Story of Buddha, Wisdom Publications, 1984.

Lark, Liz, and Ansari, Mark, Yoga for Beginners, Newleaf, 1988.

Mainland, Pauline, A Parade of Yoga Animals, Element, 1998.

Mercer, Joyce, The Complete Edition of Andersen and Grimm, Hutchinson.

Hugh, Angela, Island of the Children: An Anthology of Children's Poems, Orchard, 1987.
(Judith Nicholls' excerpts, page 86)

O'Neill, Amanda, I Wonder Why Snakes Shed Their Skin, Kingfisher, 1996.

Saint-Exupery, Antoine de, and Howard, Richard, translator, The Little Prince, Mammoth, 2000.

Snazaroo, First Faces: Facepainting, Kingfisher, 1995.

Stewart, Mary, and Phillips, Kathy, Yoga for Children, Websters, 1992.

Stukin, Stacie, 'How Yoga Helps Kids Become Better Learners', Yoga Journal, November 2001.

Tagore, Rabindranath, Particles, Jottings, Sparks, Angel Books, 2001.

Tolstoy, Leo, and Sekirin, Peter, translator, A Calendar of Wisdom, Hodder & Stoughton, 1998.

Wilde, Oscar, The Happy Prince, Puffin, 1962.

Williams, Margery, The Velveteen Rabbit, Mammoth, 1989.

INDEX

Main references to postures are in italics.

ACKNOWLEDGMENTS

Thanks to the Bihar School of Yoga, Mungar, and Satyananda Paramahansa for *Yoga Education for Children;* Clare Park for photography; Panni Bharti for face painting and inspiration; Maria at Yogahome; Robin Catto at Triyoga; and Erika. Many thanks also go to all the children who participated in the book and provided the illustrations used throughout: Amber Devetta, Ben Holmes, Charlotte Monguel, Daniel Holmes, Dominic Sedgwick, Ganga, Hannah Porter, Isabella MacKenzie, Jemima Williams, Kailash, Kieran Leahy, Oliver Monguel, Pascal Sedgwick, Phoebe Davey, Sinead Leahy, Tatiana Dyer, William Bishop, and to Panni and Mooe for their advice.

Yoga mats supplied by Yoga-Mad. Visit www.yogamad.com or call 01386 555 955 for information.

Jewellery featured throughout made by Dominic and Pascal Sedgwick.